WHAT IF IT WAS THAT

EASY?

HOW TO HEAL YOU & YOUR HOME

HOW EARTH'S ENERGIES MAY BE
AFFECTING YOUR LIFE

BY NICKY CROCKER

Illustrations by Courtney Croad

DEDICATION

I'd like to dedicate this book to all my wonderful
new friends (previously clients) who were wise enough to
listen to their gut!

Thank you!

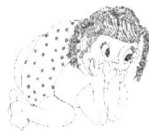

Nicky Crocker

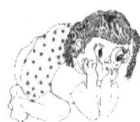

CONTENTS

Chapter One: *Page 1*

- What is Geopathic Stress?
- And why do you need to know about it?
- Six Stages of Geopathic Stress:
- **One**: First Stage, Negative Sensations
- **Two**: Negative Emotions and Sleep Disorders
- **Three**: Stress Hormone
- **Four**: Digestive System Disorder
- **Five**: Brain Damage
- **Six**: Most serious Stage, Immune damage & Chronic ill health.

Chapter Two: *Page 30*

- How could it affect my family and me?
- Relationship Issues
- Heart Issues
- Autoimmune Disease

Chapter Three: *Page 49*

- What else is affected?
- Animals & Plants?
- Animals that LIKE it
- Animals that DON'T
- Plants that LIKE it
- Plants that DON'T
- Also Caged Animals

Chapter Four: *Page 58*

- If GS is always there, then how can you be safe?
- How are you going to see it? –

Chapter Five: *Page 78*

- Why didn't you know about this before?

Chapter Six: *Page 88*

- Difference between Geomancy and Fung Shui

Chapter Seven: *Page 93*

Case studies from Allergies to Bedwetting & Cancer to Weight-gain

- Allergies
- Arthritis
- Aggression & Sudden Irritability
- Baby crying a lot – Won't Settle
- Bed Wetting
- Cancer
- Case Study I - Victoria
- Case Study II
- Child Leukemia
- Crohns
- CFS Chronic Fatigue Syndrome
- Diarrhea or Constipation

- Depression
- Dizziness/Nausea
- Eczema/Psoriasis
- Grinding teeth
- Headaches/Migraines
- IBS Irritable Bowel Syndrome
- ADHD & Learning difficulties
- Lack of Energy
- High or Low blood pressure
- Miscarriage/Cot death/ SIDS
- Sleep Disorders
- Stomach Ulcers
- Uneasy Feeling / Hot or Cold
- Weight gain or Loss

Everything from Headaches to Cancer: *Page 142*

What others have to say? *Page 147*

Chapter Eight: *Page 155*

- How do I FEEL this Energy? - A guide to dowse
- Tools:
- How to make 'L' Rods
- Plastic Rods
- Pendulum
- How to use your body

- **How to dowse 'Nicky Style'**: *Page 159*

Chapter Nine: *Page 173*

Dowsing Tests and Exercises - A fun way to explore this phenomenon

- House and Office dowsing
- Earth Grids

- **What else is dowsing good for?** *Page 179*

Chapter Ten: *Page 184*

- What else can help?
- Energy Bombs™, Crystals etc.

Chapter Eleven: *Page 190*

- Can YOU be your own House Doctor?
- What to look for - The power within!

Frequently Asked Questions: *Page 197*

About the Author: *Page 201*

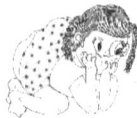

FOREWORD

What if it was that EASY? How to heal YOU and YOUR home?

Nicky Crocker is doing outstanding work helping people create healthier home environments, which leads to more positive wellbeing and quality of life.

This book will help people make wiser lifestyle and health choices and this information is long overdue for the general public.

Nicky has helped me personally with a geopathic problem in my own home especially in my bedroom. By shifting my bed my sleep improved dramatically and chronic pain in my feet reduced overnight. She has also improved the quality of our clinic environment. We shifted furniture in our clinic rooms including patient beds.

Our clients have had excellent results from Nicky's work and I recommend Nicky for her broad knowledge of what is required for a healthy home or work space and the compassion she shows for helping people.

John Coombs - Director

Global Health Clinics

A NOTE TO READERS

My book "What if it was that easy" is exactly that.

A question to yourself, to ask your body. What if my health or the health of my children and family is directly related to where we spend time 'stationary'?

What if it was that easy?

What if the place you choose to put your bed in your home, or are forced to put it because of the way the house was built, or the way your parents put your bed, was relevant to the state of your health when you were growing up?

What if it was that easy?

What if the desk you chose at work or was told to sit at, or indeed stand at all day in the same location, is in the wrong place according to these Earth Energies, and could be affecting your health?

Just because something is simple or easy, doesn't mean it can't be true.

Think about it, the significant time we spend stationary is while we are in bed, on the couch, or at our desk, and these are the times when our body is in direct alignment with the earth. Therefore if there was a 'frequency' or energy coming up from the Earth, and there is, it would be these times that you could be affected by it.

Therefore that magnetic field around earth (Schumann

resonance 7.83htz, more about this later in the book) that vibrates at a slightly higher frequency than is healthy for us, has a chance to irritate us.

You have all sat in a chair or been still in your bed, or at work, and felt tingles or a hot or cold sensation that may have given you a headache or even worse.

You have walked into a room and felt like someone was behind you. This can also be explained as this energy. Occasionally it may not be, but when you consider how many magnetic fields there are around the earth, no one has ever missed them.

In fact you walk through them every day, somewhere in your daily routine. If you spend a lot of time stationary, and on one of them, it is likely to attack your immune system and affect your health.

You don't want to be stationary on them. This book is to help you recognize and understand them.

This to make you AWARE not SCARE!

WHAT IF IT WAS THAT EASY?

ACKNOWLEDGEMENTS

To my husband Ray for all the times he has listened to my many ideas and patiently accepted them.

To my children Ashleigh and Benjamin who's experiences growing up helped me understand this phenomenon.

To Eric who first helped me understand over 20 years ago Earth's energies and how it was affecting my health and the health of others.

To all my clients, family and friends, who have let me practice and learn about this amazing subject and believed in me enough to try the simple things I have suggested which has made a difference in their lives.

To the Mentors and Geomancers around the world I have studied and trained with over the years who's knowledge and experiences I have taken to heart and learnt from.

…and a very very special thank you to Cheyney for the cover and Courtney Croad who did all the illustrations for my book. I love your imagination and wish you every success for your future artistic ventures.

I thank you forever

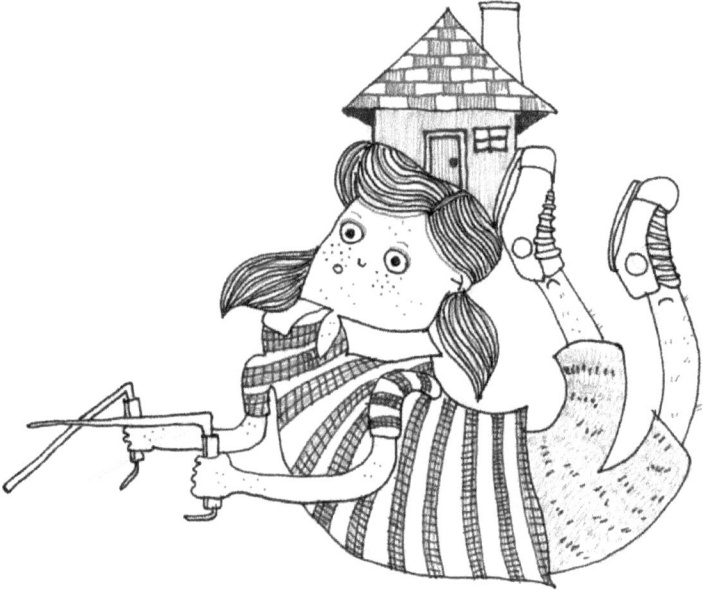

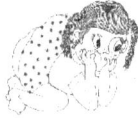

1 CHAPTER ONE

WHAT IS GEOPATHIC STRESS (GS)?
AND
WHY DO YOU NEED TO KNOW ABOUT IT?

Ok, I'm guessing you've either never heard of Geopathic Stress, or if you have, want to know more about this exciting phenomenon known as Geopathic Stress or Noxious Earth Energy, and how it can affect you in your home or office.

Or you picked up the wrong book and now you're interested hehe!

Either way this book is about to blow your mind, not literally but it is a better way of finding out about this subject than I did 20 years ago, when I was told that I was being affected by Geopathic Stress and my body was like a 100 year old fungus, Eeewwww!

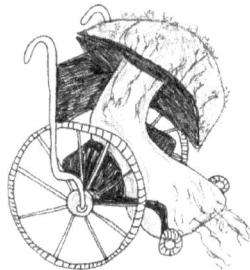

1

So to start with and to get the 'official' explanations out of the way, here are a few of the meanings I have found over the years, but all say a similar thing!

Geopathic Stress: Is natural radiation that rises up through the earth and becomes distorted by weak electro-magnetic fields, created by subterranean running water, certain mineral concentrations, fault lines, and underground cavities. *(Wikipedia)*

Geopathic Stress: Negative health effects on the body caused by geomagnetic frequency. (Google)

Geopathic: (comparative more geopathic, superlative most geopathic) 1. Relating to the theory that natural irregularities in the earth's magnetic field can be intensified by power lines, underground pipelines, and other natural and man-made features such that a stress field harmful to human health and well-being is created. *(Wiktionary)*

Geopathic Stress: (also known as geostress) is a form of trauma caused by disturbed or irregular energies within the earth's mantle. The Earth is surrounded by an energy grid, which contains and transmits vital forces. This grid is essential to life, and is part of the background radiation, which supports life. However, this energetic grid can become traumatized and the energies, which it contains and emanates, can become harmful to life, for us as humans but also impacts plants and animals. *(Alex Stark www.alexstark.com ref)*

<u>Geopathic Stress:</u> has been implicated in a number of undesirable effects to human health, from simple conditions such as sleeplessness or confusion to highly dangerous ones such as cancer, decreased fertility, and autoimmune dysfunction. *(Alex Stark <u>www.alexstark.com</u> ref)*

In Europe it is sometimes called Radiesthesia; this word was first coined in 1935 and has a Latin heritage.

The energy grids are known as Hartmann, Curry, Schumann, named after the scientist that discovered them. But on top of these above, the movement of underground water, (which of course does not go in a nice neat pattern like Hartmann and Curry grids), can cause Geopathic Stress. Just like rivers on the surface they move all over the place therefore this makes it difficult to detect and identify.

Well there's the official explanation, or some of them:

SO WHY DO YOU NEED TO KNOW ABOUT THIS?

Just because you have never heard of something or perhaps you may have heard of it, but not really taken much notice, that doesn't mean it's not time to listen to something new.

Or maybe some 'woo woo lady or man' once told you something about it, but you figured it was not something you were really interested in, so switched off.

NOW IT'S TIME TO PAY ATTENTION.

You could be making your life a lot harder and less healthy by NOT knowing about Geopathic Stress.

Generally I have found in the past around 90% of people have never heard of it, but when I explain it they usually 'get it' as it resonates in their 'truth' system.

Isn't life about being informed?

Yes of course it is you say, so how did you not know about this before today?

Knowledge is power? So let's give you some of that power!

If it was that important shouldn't it be taught in school?

Well that's my next adventure. I'll start with you first and then work towards that.

Ok, so how can this Geopathic Stress affect you?

How can energy from some water that is trapped deep under the crust of the earth hurt me where I sleep in my bed you may ask. How is it I can be completely oblivious to that underground water or any other Noxious Earth Energy that may be creeping around my room, yet it can affect me and even make me sick, really sick? If I can't see it, or feel it then how can it hurt me right?

So many questions, but we'll get to those answers shortly with lots of examples you may relate to.

You CAN feel it! Or at least be affected by it!

Have you ever walked into a room and felt a chill, and it's been a warm day? Or you have felt a warm feeling when it had been a cool day?

Have you felt tingles or pins and needles when you are sleeping or sitting in a certain location?

Have you ever felt uncomfortable in a certain chair or seat at work or at home and you just thought it was not a comfy chair?

Have you ever been to the theatre or the movies and had your legs tingle the whole time you were sitting there and just thought your shoes were too tight?

Funnily that did happen to me, and I was sure it was my boots, but when I took them off, my legs still tingled and were completely uncomfortable. Then I couldn't get my boots back on. Epic Fail.

Or have you got a headache or neck ache when you have sat down to dinner at restaurant, or even at home.

Have you ever started getting backache when sitting at your desk at work when you only just sat down? Or felt that someone was watching over your shoulder when you know there was no one there?

Or felt agitated in certain places quite quickly.

5

There are many symptoms that you may recognize that I've listed below:

- ✓ Drowsiness,

- ✓ Dizziness,

- ✓ Weakness,

- ✓ Headaches,

- ✓ Irritability,

- ✓ Fatigue, Lethargy

- ✓ Feeling depressed,

- ✓ Anxiety,

- ✓ Lack of appetite in the morning,

- ✓ Accelerated heartbeat,

- ✓ Increased blood sugar levels,

- ✓ And these are to name just a few.

Yes, I've experienced a few of these you say, who hasn't? Or maybe you know someone that does, and you may be thinking how can my bed or favourite chair at home, or my office desk position be causing these symptoms?

How on earth can underground water or whatever this 'energy' is be causing my headaches - right?

Come on, when I go to the beach or anywhere near the water, it makes my headaches go away and it makes me feel great, or if I have a headache a glass of water helps it, so that can't be it - Can it?

What if it was that easy?

If it was that easy then why haven't I heard about this before?

Why didn't my parents tell me this stuff?

Why why why?

Ok enough already, give me more.

I remember my Granddad finding water on the farm when I was young, but that was for a water well so he could irrigate the farm and feed the stock, not so he could find somewhere safe to sleep. Although I do remember him telling me stories about watching where the sheep and cattle slept, and that is where they would build their new homes.

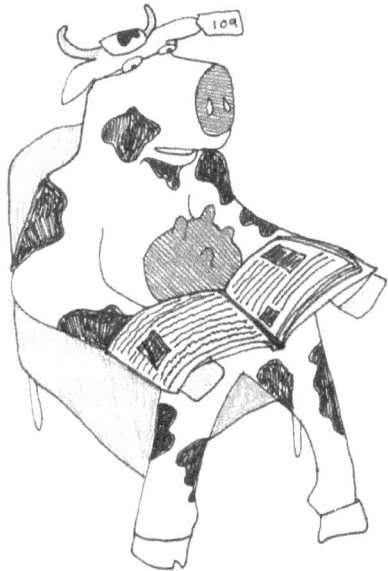

Was that it?

Did the sheep and cattle know something we didn't?

Are they really more intelligent than us?

Or are they just more sensitive at detecting it?

You're right; they're more sensitive, but not necessarily more sensitive than human beings. It's just they are not listening to iPods, or headphones connected to our phones, and being influenced by what we see on television, or read, or hear and what we have been taught verbatim at school for years and years.

They sense something that doesn't 'feel' right so they keep away from it. Simple – right?

Then why can't we do that?

The simple answer is we can! It's just that years and years of 'conditioning' to think that those feelings are something else. Like those headaches are because we have not drunk enough water (and that maybe the case) or we drank too much, or not enough coffee, or too much, or we have taken too many painkillers and now we have just got used to them.

There are many other reasonable answers that we have been told for years and years, and many could be accurate but what if that's not the answer in YOUR situation?

Did anyone ever tell you if you are sitting, standing, or lying in the wrong position and it could be detrimentally affecting your health?

And by that I mean one that is being affected by this Noxious Earth energy, called Geopathic Stress.

The seat you chose at work or the bed you chose (or were given by parents who didn't know) could be the cause of your bad health?

Could it be that easy? What if it was?

Did they have the same level of disease and health issues 100 or more years ago when they had more of a luxury to choose where they put their homes? These days we are living in more

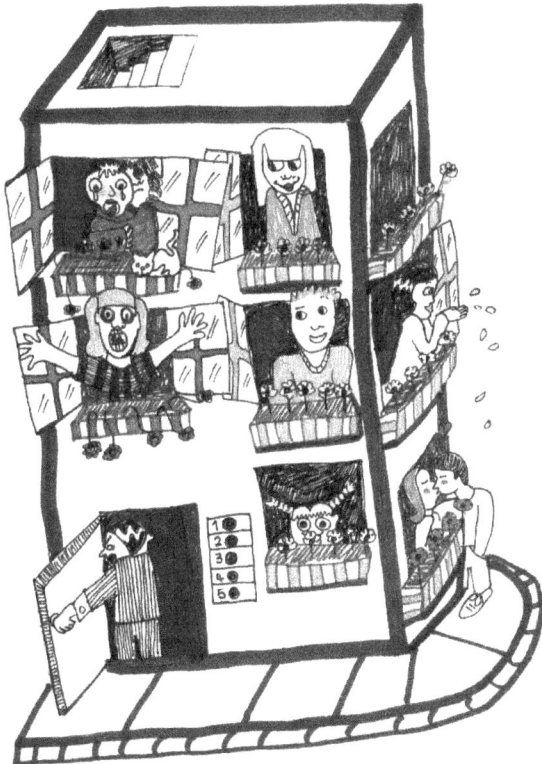

condensed areas, living on top of each other.

We build apartment buildings with the same or similar floor plans and wonder why we have sick building syndromes. Is this because the same floor plans and bedroom layouts are all placed in the same position on the land, and these 'energies' come from deep within the surface of the earth and travel up through the layers and then continue up through the concrete and steel and integrity of the apartment buildings.

Sadly if a noxious energy line is running right through the middle of the floor plan where the bedrooms are, and a 'built-in' wardrobe has been included, and there really is only one position for the bed to go, chances are you are going to be affected by this energy.

How do we protect ourselves?

How do you make sure that some of the negative effects of Geopathic Stress won't make you sick?

How would you like to learn how to do it yourself?

Well now you can, and this is in more detail later in chapter eight on 'How to Dowse'!

There are six stages of Geopathic Stress. There are probably many more, but to simplify them into 6 stages, makes you realize how the symptoms may be affecting you and my goal is to get people to be aware in the earlier stages and have their homes tested (or test themselves, with the abilities taught later in the book), certainly before they get to stages 5 or 6.

There are six stages of Geopathic Stress (GS)

STAGE ONE:

This changes from person to person and can occur within a few hours up to several weeks.

Most people don't pay much attention and don't even seek medical advice. It may represent as a Negative feeling or Sensation. Some won't recover from a common illness, or injury. You may not get over the flu or have symptoms that hang around longer than they should. This is the stage where there are no symptoms but the manifestation of neurotransmitter imbalance has already occurred.

Geopathic Stress inhibits neurotransmitters, especially serotonin, which in this stage can lead to mood dysfunction and apathy. Most people do not recognize these feelings as being associated with any 'external' thing; so avoid doing something as simple as checking for GS and moving away from it.

If you moved away from it, the symptoms and feelings can be permanently eliminated.

If you stay there, it will develop into stage two.

Some symptoms you may recognize:

- ✓ Unpleasant sensations
- ✓ Mood disorders

11

- ✓ Apathy
- ✓ Flabbiness
- ✓ Worry
- ✓ Unreasonable sadness

Feeling uncomfortable in your bed, favourite armchair or workplace without any particular reason.

STAGE TWO: Sleep Disorders & Negative Emotions

This stage can occur within a few days or several months. It is typically characterized by continued neurotransmitter imbalances, which lead to two types of symptoms, Sleep Disorders and Negative Emotional Effects.

Sleep Disorders: Constant inhibition of neurotransmitters (a chemical by which a nerve cell communicates with another nerve cell or muscle) such as serotonin, GABA (Gama Amino Butyric Acid) and norepinephrine (or noradrenaline, a hormone secreted by the adrenal medulla, increasing blood pressure and heart rate) can lead to Insomnia, waking up tired, and restless sleep.

These symptoms can seriously disrupt people's life and can lead to dizziness, weakness and drowsiness.

It can also cause irritability, lack of appetite in the morning, headaches, fatigue etc. All these symptoms are not constant however you could experience them often.

Yet still it is not enough to make you think you need to go to the Doctor. If you did the Doctor would probably not find anything wrong with your health and recommend rest, normal sleep and avoid stress.

The other side of this is:

Negative Emotions:

This will happen when you have a decrease in serotonin or GABA and can cause Negative emotions to occur constantly.

You will have feelings of Depression, Anxiety, Helplessness and Impending doom. Of course these can have a great effect on humans and will affect their lifestyles. It will affect work relationships and create family conflicts. Some researchers believe that the fact you don't express these negative emotions and can be tied to specific illnesses and can increase the risk of illness as it weakens the body. With a virus or other medical condition, negative emotions can indeed affect the course of the illness and the recovery process. As soon as Geopathic Stress gets to the point where the human body's hormones get involved, the 2nd stage gradually transitions into stage 3. Some of the symptoms you may experience at this stage:

- ✓ Feeling cold or shivering in bed

- ✓ Anxiety

- ✓ Lack of appetite in the morning

- ✓ Sleep disorders

- ✓ Difficulty falling asleep

- ✓ Impending doom

- ✓ Drowsiness

- ✓ Weakness

- ✓ Headaches

- ✓ Irritability

- ✓ Difficulty staying awake

- ✓ Waking frequently

- ✓ Nightmares

- ✓ Fatigue

- ✓ Feeling depressed

- ✓ Night sweats

STAGE THREE:

Stress Hormone Stage:

This is long one but very important. This is when major symptoms occur; these can happen in a few months or several years.

These symptoms can remain for a long time, but once the cause

of the Geopathic threat is avoided, the body function and health conditions usually go back to normal.

How good is that!

During the few months and years GS has a negative influence on the body, serious threats may occur to your physical and mental health. The body starts to actively respond to the natural radiation threat. The human body tries to defend itself and do whatever needs to be done to protect the brain and other organs.

The hypothalamus sends signals to the sympathetic nervous system. The sympathetic system becomes activated in response to that threat. Also the HPA system triggers the production and release of the stress hormone cortisol.

Cortisol is very important in the marshaling system throughout the body, including the heart, lungs, circulation, metabolism, and immune system. The HBA system also releases certain neurotransmitters (catecholamines, which are the sympathomimetic 'fight-or-flight' hormones that are released by the adrenal glands in response to stress), dopamine, norepinephrine, and epinephrine.

Geopathic Stress leads to sexual dysfunction, increases the likelihood of illness, and often the manifestation of skin ailments. Epinephrine (adrenalin) raises the heart rate, breathing rate, blood pressure, and the amount of sugar in the blood.

This can lead to symptoms including, fatigue and weakness, muscle and bone loss, moodiness or depression, hormone imbalance, and suppression of the immune system.

If Geopathic Stress never shuts off, i.e. you are sleeping for 6-8 hours a night and also working on a GS zone, then these stress hormones produce feelings of anxiety and helplessness.

Over-sensitivity to Geopathic Stress has been linked with severe depression, because depressed people have a harder time adapting to the negative side effects of cortisol (stress hormone).

Excessive amounts of cortisol can cause sleep disturbances, loss of sex drive, and lack of interest in sex. Depression and anxiety may contribute to illness and this may cause people to be depressed or anxious.

Tense muscles can cause headaches and neck pain.

In this stage (3), if you eliminate Geopathic zones, they will have no further adverse health and emotional conditions. In short bursts, elevated adrenalin is not damaging or dangerous. In fact, that is what it is designed to do.

But when sustained at high levels over a period of time, it can be very harmful. Such long-term over-arousal and excessive flow of this hormone will eventually lead to physiological and psychological distress.

In short, look out for these symptoms in yourself or your friends and if you think there might be a problem, it is very simple to get it checked by a dowser or Geomancer.

(Or later learn how to dowse yourself)

Some of the symptoms you may experience in this stage are:

- ✓ Accelerated human heartbeat
- ✓ Increased breathing rate
- ✓ Increased blood sugar
- ✓ Hypertension
- ✓ Depression
- ✓ Muscle cramps tension, pain
- ✓ Numbness in arms and legs
- ✓ Tingling in arms and legs
- ✓ Neck pain
- ✓ Anxiety
- ✓ Loss of sex drive
- ✓ Lack of interest in sex
- ✓ Helplessness
- ✓ Temporary impotence
- ✓ Migraine Headaches.

STAGE FOUR:

Digestive System Disorder.

It takes one to three years for symptoms to occur in this stage. If GS is not detected for this many years, physical changes respond to these natural threats and the body can't cope with these negative effects.

The human organism tries to adapt to Geopathic Stress by producing and activating more hormones, increasing blood pressure, and increasing blood sugar levels to sustain energy. The result is, it changes the body's energy reserves.

Geopathic Stress constantly influences the human body, by gradually weakening the internal organs, upsetting homeostasis (an ideal or virtual state of equilibrium, in which all body systems are working and interacting) leaving humans vulnerable to diseases.

GS affects all parts of the body, including the digestive system. Diseases of the stomach and intestines are often linked to GS because the blood has to leave these organs and move to muscles.

Prolonged Geopathic Stress can disrupt the digestive system, irritating the large intestine and causing diarrhoea, constipation, cramping and bloating. It's common to have a stomach ache. This happens because stress hormones slow the release of stomach acid and the emptying of the stomach.

The same hormones also stimulate the colon, which controls speed of the passage of its contents. Geopathic Stress may predispose some people to ulcers or sustain existing ulcers. Irritable Bowel Syndrome (spastic colon) is strongly related to Geopathic Stress.

This hormone can increase appetite and cause weight gain. To reiterate, chronically elevated cortisol (I talked about this in Stage 2 and 3) levels contribute to the accumulation of abdominal fat, and make it very difficult to counteract tension and therefore you gain weight.

Weight gain can occur even with a healthy diet in people exposed to Geopathic Stress. The release of cortisol appears to promote abnormal fat, and may be a primary connection between Geopathic Stress and weight gain in such people.

In rare cases, Geopathic Stress may trigger hyperactivity of the thyroid gland. This stimulates appetite but can cause the body to burn up calories at a faster rate, therefore people lose weight.

Cortisol and DHEA (short for dehydroepiandrosterone, is a hormone that's produced in the body and is converted into male and female hormones) work as a team to get people through prolonged Geopathic Stress effects.

DHEA is the most abundant hormone in the bloodstream. It seems to balance the effects of cortisol by improving the body's ability to cope with Geopathic Stress. DHEA also provides the raw material for the production of many other hormones including oestrogen, progesterone, and testosterone.

Clinical studies suggest the DHEA can boost energy levels and reduce body fat, but when they are straining and being attacked by Geopathic Stress it can contribute to fatigue, bone loss, loss of muscle mass, decreased sex drive, and impaired immune function. This can have a serious effect on the human organism and can lead to many health and mental problems, including memory impairment, lack of energy, heart and vessel diseases, depression, immune system suppression, and even increased susceptibility to stroke and cancer.

But the good news is, if you move off Geopathic Stress zones, your system can then have the chance to immediately start to repair.

Symptoms can subside and eventually disappear. It takes around 6-8 weeks to clear GS out of your system, avoiding it for the majority of times you spend stationary.

Some of the symptoms of this stage:

- ✓ Diarrhoea
- ✓ Constipation
- ✓ Cramping
- ✓ Bloating
- ✓ IBS - Irritable Bowel Syndrome
- ✓ Increased Appetite

- ✓ Weight Gain
- ✓ Abdominal Fat
- ✓ Weight Loss
- ✓ Fatigue
- ✓ Bone Loss
- ✓ Loss of Muscle mass
- ✓ Decreased Sex Drive
- ✓ Impaired Immune Function

STAGE FIVE:

The Brain Damage Stage

In this stage, symptoms can occur within 3-5 years. The body has run out of its reserve of body energy and immunity. Mental, physical and emotional resources suffer heavily.

Instead of shutting off once the crisis is over, the process continues, with the hypothalamus continuing to signal the adrenals to produce cortisol (remember I told you about this in the previous stages). The increased cortisol production exhausts the stress mechanism, leading to chronic fatigue and anxiety. Cortisol also interferes with serotonin activity, furthering the depressive effect. Prolonged high cortisol levels lead to high blood sugar that may develop into diabetes.

Diabetes disrupts the body's mechanism for the moving glucose out of the bloodstream and using it in cells.

As a result, levels of blood glucose stay excessively high, leading to serious complications over time.

The adrenals become depleted, leading to decreased Geopathic Stress tolerance, progressive mental and physical exhaustion, illness and collapse.

As soon as the Geopathic Stress reaches the exhaustion point, it starts to affect the major organs and systems in the human body.

Damaged functions include the cardiovascular and respiratory systems, kidney, muscles, joints and more importantly the immune system. Then individuals become more susceptible to infections, both minor and major. Very often a person in middle age will think that this is a sign of premature ageing, but examining the problem in more depth, it is likely the person has lived with Geopathic Stress for a long time. A few years' overreaction to Geopathic Stress overloads the brain with powerful hormones that are intended only for short-term duty in emergency situations.

The cumulative effect is damage of the brain cells.

Catecholamine suppresses activity in areas at the front of the brain concerned with memory, concentration, inhibition, and rational thought. Stress hormones divert blood glucose from the brain, and energy to the hypothalamus is diminished.

The typical victim of long term Geopathic Stress complains of the following:

Loss of concentration at work and at home, learning problems, inappropriate responses to major changes in life situations, inability to sit for very long, behaviour problems, aggression, problems staying calm, insecurity, self-confidence problems, panic attacks, and emotional problems (anxieties, depression, and exhaustion).

Symptoms of the Fifth Stage:

- ✓ Diabetes
- ✓ Inability to heal
- ✓ Difficulty Concentrating
- ✓ Learning problems
- ✓ Behaviour problems
- ✓ Aggression
- ✓ Memory Problems
- ✓ Lack of interest in doing something
- ✓ Decision-making problems
- ✓ Inadequate responses to major changes in life situations
- ✓ ADD (Attention Deficit Disorder)
- ✓ Chronic Fatigue

Now the last and most Serious STAGE SIX:

In this stage, symptoms can occur with 5 years or more. This stage is associated with a high risk for serious cardiac events and complete suppression of the immune system.

Stress hormones that act on the heart, blood vessels, and the lungs may contribute to heart diseases, high blood pressure and asthma.

Recent research has made it very clear that hyper-arousal of the adrenal system is the essential causative factor in coronary and arterial diseases. The chronic increased flow of adrenalin and cortisol and sympathetic nervous system activities may negatively affect the heart in several ways.

1. Increases the pumping action of the heart and causes the arteries to constrict, thereby posing a risk for blocking blood flow the heart.

2. Emotional effects during Geopathic Stress alter the heart rhythms and pose a risk for serious arrhythmia in people with existing heart rhythm disturbances.

3. Causes blood to become thicker increasing the likelihood of artery-clogging blood clots.

4. An increase in the production of blood cholesterol.

5. A decrease in the body's ability to remove cholesterol.

6. Causes people who have relatively low levels of the neurotransmitter serotonin to produce more of certain immune proteins (called cytokines), which in high amounts causes inflammation and damage to cells including possibly heart cells.

Cortisol levels also appear to play a role in the accumulation of abdominal fat, which give people an 'apple' shape. People with apple body shapes have a higher risk of heart diseases than do people with 'pear' body shapes, where weight is more concentrated in the hips.

These effects can lead to great risk factors for heart attack, heart rhythm abnormalities and stroke. Continually high cortisol levels lead to suppression of the immune system through increased production of interleukin-6 (an immune system messenger).

Research's findings indicate that prolonged Geopathic Stress and depression have a negative effect on the immune system. Also, adrenal exhaustion, which occurs at this stage, involves a depletion of energy reserves and loss of resilience.

The body's energy reserves are exhausted, and resistance to Geopathic Stress may gradually reduce, or may collapse quickly. This means the immune system and the body's ability to resist disease may be almost totally eliminated. The body runs out of the immunity to fight disease, and breakdown will occur.

Thereby reduced immunity makes the body more susceptible to everything from cold and flu to cancer.

Geopathic Stress appears to blunt the immune response and increases the risk of infection.

A number of studies have shown that subjects under Geopathic Stress have low white blood cell counts and are vulnerable to infections and diseases.

Long-term exposure to Geopathic zones can cause bronchial asthma. Rheumatoid arthritis also can be caused by an aberration of the body's immune defence mechanism, possibly overactive B cells (a type of white blood cell called a B-lymphocyte that produce antibodies) or defective regulation by T cells. (a type of blood cell that protects the body from infection).

Geopathic Stress has been implicated in increasing the risk for periodontal disease, which is disease in the gums that can cause tooth loss.

This stage of Geopathic Stress can worsen many skin conditions such as psoriasis, eczema, hives and acne. Thereby all those diseases are connected to the immune suppression process, which very often can lead people to die from such diseases as cancer, pneumonia, coronary disease, or infection. The death does not come from Geopathic Stress itself.

The human organism loses all its resistance in its effort to ward off the prolonged effects of Geopathic Stress.

Symptoms of Stage Six

- ✓ Cancer
- ✓ Cardiovascular diseases
- ✓ Heart attack
- ✓ Heart attack
- ✓ Arthritis
- ✓ Kidney Disorders
- ✓ Allergies
- ✓ Skin Diseases
- ✓ Bronchial Asthma
- ✓ Stroke
- ✓ Infertility and miscarriages

How many of these can you tick off?

I'm sure you are saying but these are all the chronic illnesses that people have, how can Geopathic Stress cause these too? Let me reiterate, GS does NOT CAUSE any of these illnesses or Dis-Ease.

We need these frequencies of energy for life, as we know it. Just like the sun, we cannot live without it, but if you lay out in the sun to long, you will get burnt. Therefore that is not good.

It is the same with the magnetic fields of earth and the stress caused by underground water, i.e. Geopathic Stress. We need them, but we don't want to be on them for long periods of time.

What this energy does is vibrates at a frequency that is way above a healthy bodily frequency, (which is the Schumann resonance 7.83htz) and if it is crossing a certain part of your body (or your whole body), then all the cells in that part of your body won't cope and your immune system will slowly get lowered, depending on what else is going on in your life to a point it will struggle to cope. i.e. these illnesses and dis-ease will attack.

The 'lines' of energy caused by either the magnetic fields or underground water, vary considerably from around 29-30 cm, up to half a metre, and occasionally even wider.

For underground water, just like the rivers and streams on the surface of the earth, they move all over the place and don't go in straight lines like the Earth's magnetic fields seem to. This makes it harder to detect and map.

The Schumann resonances (SR) are a set of spectrum peaks in the extremely low frequency (ELF) portion of the Earth's electromagnetic field spectrum. Schumann resonances are global electromagnetic resonances, generated and excited by lightning discharges in the cavity formed by the Earth's surface and the ionosphere. **note from Wikipedia*

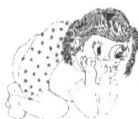

2 CHAPTER TWO
HOW COULD IT AFFECT MY FAMILY AND ME?

Ok so we have worked out what 'it' is.

Geopathic Stress is an energy that is created by underground water from deep within the surface of the earth. Also a number of other energy grids such as the Hartman, Curry, Schumann, and Ley lines. But we will go into those later in the book.

What you do need to know is that these energies are everywhere!

They have to be struck by lightning somewhere around the world so many times a second to keep them charged. Apparently there are at least 100 lightning strikes that hit the earth every second, so guess that is covered.

We need them for our very existence, but you need to be aware of where they are in your beautiful house, or workplace.

If you have just bought one, or if you have lived in the same home your whole life or even if you are only renting one, they must be checked for your own peace of mind!

Don't think that because you don't own it, it won't affect you. Who cares about if it has dry rot, or termites, or some damp issues, 'You don't own it, you'll just move if it gets too bad', right?

No, you are still 'living' in the space so you will still be being affected by this noxious earth energy.

Did the real estate agent tell you there were energy lines in this house?

Do they have to?

I don't think you would have bought it if you knew that there could be big red lines running though the bedrooms of your beautiful new house. Especially if they could affect your health.

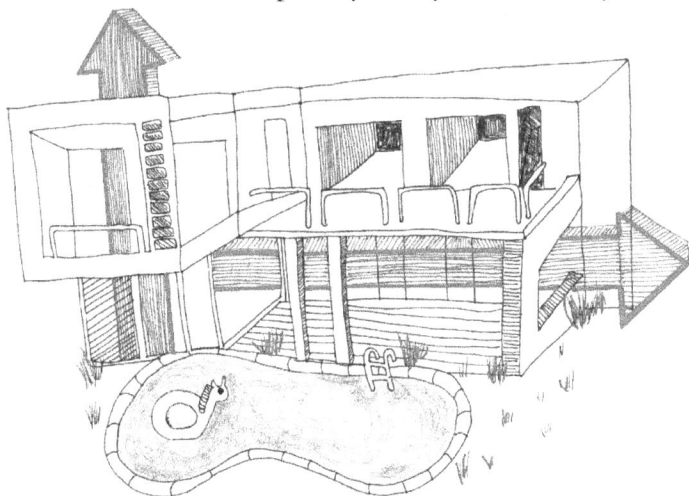

Shouldn't they (Real Estate agents) have told me, you ask?

How could they if they didn't know themselves?

Maybe they are just like you and didn't know about these Noxious Earth Energies either.

However if they (real estate agents) thought about it, they may see a pattern with some of the homes that frequently become available on the market. They call them 'divorce' houses because everyone that buys 'that house' suffers a marriage break-up within a few years and they have to sell again.

Must be an unlucky house you say!

But they sure don't want 'you' as a new buyer to know that!

Will you be scared off?

Maybe it just needs to have the building biology test done on the house and this problem could be eliminated.

When you buy a house, there are many checks you do before you sign on the dotted line, you may get a 'building inspection', checking out that the foundations are strong, and there are no unexpected surprises.

Sadly, normally a building inspection does not pick up Geopathic Stress or Noxious Earth Energy.

Believe me it is far more important than finding out if you have termites or dry rot? Oh and by the way, chances are if you do, you will have bad Geopathic Stress.

You can replace a few boards or spray for termites.

Geopathic Stress is not so easy to remove.

Especially if it is running directly through the middle of the bedroom where you would put a bed and your body or worse your child's.

Don't let there be a monster under your bed.

Also don't let that 'clear' wall where you might add a wardrobe, be the best wall to put your bed!

Another scenario is, homes where one person in the house has developed cancer and/or sadly died. They (Real Estate agents) would not want to pass on that information as it may dissuade you from buying or moving in.

However these are the questions you must ask before you think of buying or even renting a home. You **must** know the history.

Don't be afraid of the answer because it can be changed.

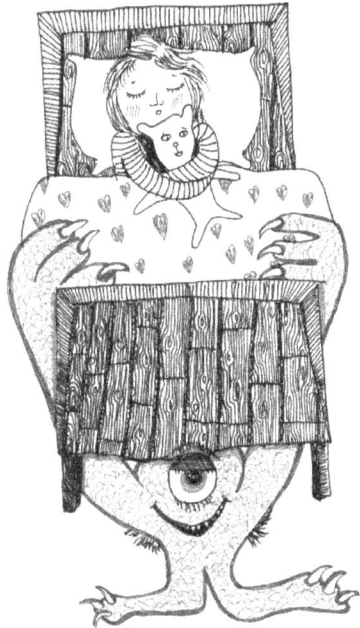

I had a friend who sadly rang me to say his Mum had been diagnosed with cancer, and he of course was devastated. About one month later he rang back to tell me that his Dad had also been diagnosed with cancer. I asked him to ask his parents if they knew the history of the house and the previous owners.

My friend rang me back 20 minutes later to say the previous owners that had lived in the house before his parents moved in 5 years earlier, had both died of, yes you guessed it, Cancer.

Believe it or not, they both had the same cancer in the same parts of their bodies as his parents.

Could it be the location of the bed? Exactly where the GS came through the bed! Coincidence? Or just bad luck?

Why did they not ask the history of the house before they moved in? No one ever suggested this was something you asked when moving into a new property? Let alone a house you were buying. Who cares what the previous owners did. This is our new house and we are not them, right?

They were probably just so excited to get a unit in this sought after location. At no point did they think that their new house was going to be the death of them!

Why did this happen? Would a different bed position have made a difference? Possibly!

But with statistics from studies done all over the world from Germany to Canada, and USA to UK, they show that GS and Cancer are linked at a rate of around 95% of cases to be found where the person was sleeping in their beds.

They say that 'Geopathic Stress does not cause cancer, but in every case of cancer, we have found Geopathic Stress to be present'!

This is why a simple Geomancy Test would have identified any possible Noxious Earth Energy in the home, allowing them to make an educated decision.

- o   Was the bedroom layout going to work that way?

- o   Do we need to move the beds to avoid the noxious earth energy?

- o   Can we live with the bed in that position?

- o   How much is our health worth?

Good Health makes life a lot easier…and cheaper!

These are simple questions to ask that could have a huge implication on your future good health.

A very quick and relatively easy test by a qualified dowser could answer lots of questions. (And I'm about to teach you to do it for yourself, so keep reading)

Through my work over the last 20 years or more detecting Geopathic Stress in homes and work places, I have become very sensitive to these Noxious Earth Energies, and now when I go away or stay somewhere new, I will always dowse to make sure that the bed is in a good position.

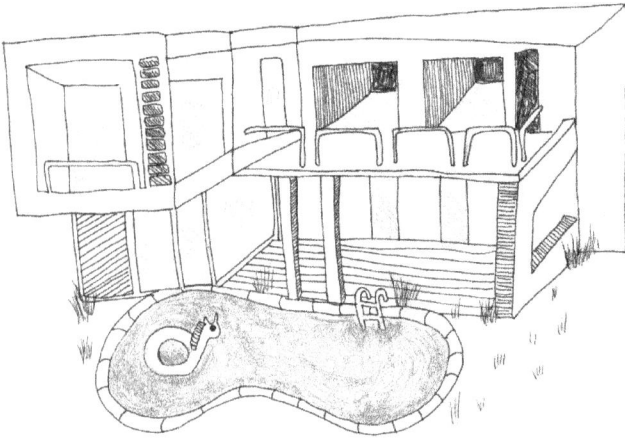

I have visited some seriously beautiful homes that you would not believe could be affected by anything 'negative'.

When a house is new and beautifully decorated, how could it possibly be bad for you? Believe me it can. We stayed recently in this home with spectacular views overlooking hills and lakes, such a beautiful setting. It had the most luxurious beds with 1000 count cotton sheets, so for sure you must have a good night sleep, right? Wrong!

My husband did (on the first night) as he chose the other side of the bed and is not normally as sensitive as I am. After retiring for the night, within 30 minutes I started to feel body irritation and an uncomfortable feeling. I immediately knew this was a very bad place to sleep. Although I had enjoyed a lovely meal with wine, and should have slept easily, I could tell I was going to be kept awake all night.

The bed was too heavy to move away from the wall and the problem energy line I was sensing, so the best and quickest option was simply to move to the other end of the bed. With my head where my feet would normally go, at the other end away from those noxious energy lines, that were crossing the pillows, I had a perfect nights sleep with no interruptions.

Funnily the next night, my husband decided to also sleep at the other end of the bed, because when I checked how he slept, he also felt the same irritation, and it had woken him up in the early hours of the morning.

Most people would have stayed there all night, eventually falling into an exhausted coma sleep, tossing and turning for the rest of the night, waking up in the morning with a headache and blaming the wine.

They would then struggle on during the day, and start to feel better later in the day when the sunshine had finally charged their body. Or the 3rd cup of coffee finally zapped their body to an, 'awake mode' and the bad nights sleep finally forgotten, only to do it all over again the next night.

Sadly there are millions and millions of people around the world who think their bad nights sleep, is due to:

- ✓ An uncomfortable bed,

- ✓ Too much food before bed,

- ✓ Too much alcohol, or not enough

- ✓ Coffee

- ✓ Kids, No kids,

- ✓ Pets,

- ✓ Too hot, too cold,

- ✓ Stress and worries of life,

- ✓ Uncomfortable pillow,

The list goes on and on.

There are many other variables that are typical symptoms of bad or interrupted sleep.   Of course the above could also be contributing factors.

Or could it be that the bed is just in the wrong position in your house?

During past World Wars they used 'Sleep Deprivation' as one of the worst tortures, yet we are unwittingly doing the same thing to ourselves.

What if it was that easy?

I remember having a conversation with a friend who confessed he was an insomniac. He never slept through the night, and this had always been the case. Well since they had lived in this house.

I asked him how he slept when was away on holiday? Realizing he had been sleeping better without snoring, he said, "That's different, I'm away on holiday! You always sleep better when you are on holiday, don't you"?

Not necessarily! I suggested that when he gets home to move his bed to the left, as I was aware of a skin cancer recently removed from the right side of his face. I believed the bed needed to move to the left away from that side. He was intrigued enough that I made him promise to try it when he returned home.

He rang me a week later to advise that he had slept through the night, every night since moving the bed. What's more, He had slept in that bed for 25 years and NEVER slept through the night! Thinking that was his normal sleep pattern, and he was just an insomniac.

How has this affected his energy levels over the years?

How has it affected the way he treats his family and staff?

Was he grumpier than usual?

Is he as healthy as he could have been if he had slept in a position that allowed him to sleep through the night, and wake in the morning feeling like he had actually had a satisfying nights sleep?

How does this problem affect your organs? When instead of resting and restoring the energy lost during waking hours, as our bodies are supposed to do, they spend the night fighting off the negative effects of this noxious earth energy. No wonder we sometimes wake up feeling tired, especially if we are sleeping in a noxiously affected area.

Could it be as easy as moving my bed?

What if it was that easy?

Then there was the young girl that after moving into their new house chose the room to the left instead of the right where her sister went. This physically and mentally affected her for the rest of her life. She had weight issues, skin allergies and learning difficulties, to name a few. Her sister had none of these. And sadly it was unwittingly her choice, as she wanted that bedroom!

Could the choice of which bed you chose (location) have possibly such a detrimental effect on your health?

Could it be possible that these Noxious Earth Energies have caused the allergies, psoriasis and asthma that have invaded her body throughout her young life?

Is the excess weight she is now carrying be the result of an inability for her body to rest and rejuvenate during the night, preventing her body fighting off Geopathic Stress and not allowing it the time to metabolize the excess calories, and making her feel lethargic.

Was that why she felt sluggish all the time? Especially when she woke in the morning?

Was that why she felt dizzy when she woke up?

Was that why she had food allergies and struggled with maintaining a healthy weight?

Can you imagine spending ten to fifteen years in a bedroom

that you knew was giving you diabetes, or causing the terrible psoriasis or eczema on your skin!

Wouldn't you want to know about this before you moved into that bedroom?

Would you stay there?

No of course you wouldn't! I suspect there is no way you would stay in a position if you could physically see these energy lines.

If you walked into that house and there was a big red line running across one corner of the room warning you to keep away from that side of the room, and then a big green line saying "put your bed here!"…

I'm guessing it would be quite obvious where you would put your bed.

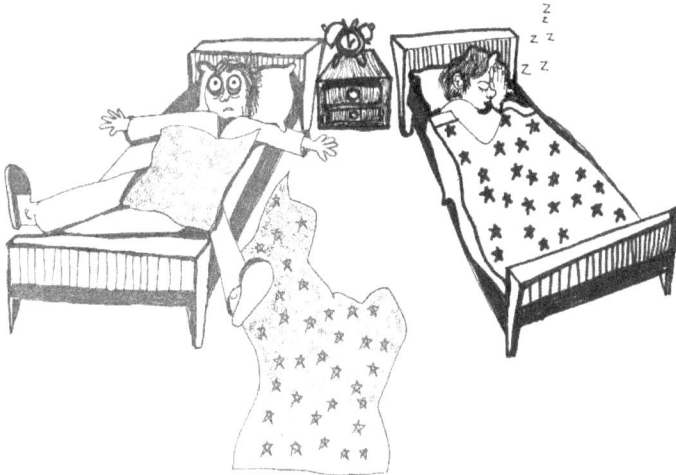

Sadly we don't have that luxury! Or do we?

What if it was that easy?

Here are some health issues that have been typically related to Geopathic Stress…

<u>RELATIONSHIP ISSUES</u>

One of my clients who ran a healing business out of her apartment, while living at the back of the premises noticed that when her new partner joined her in her new home, things started to go wrong.

He started to get angry and irritable, he was always sick and would toss and turn at night. This was not the man she had met, and it certainly wasn't what he was like before they moved in together.

He was running his business from the lounge room and dining area of the house, while she was working from the front of the house.

She had been very happy in this space on her own, but having another person living there was starting taking its toll on her.

It wasn't the fact that they were crowded together in a small one-bedroom unit, she was really happy about that.

She knew what I did with Geopathic Stress detection as I had already checked a previous home of hers, so she rang and asked me to check her new apartment.

I detected a line running through the house and sadly the 3 places her boyfriend spent the most time, his bed, couch and his seat at the dining table where he worked on his computer during the day, were all badly affected by Geopathic Stress.

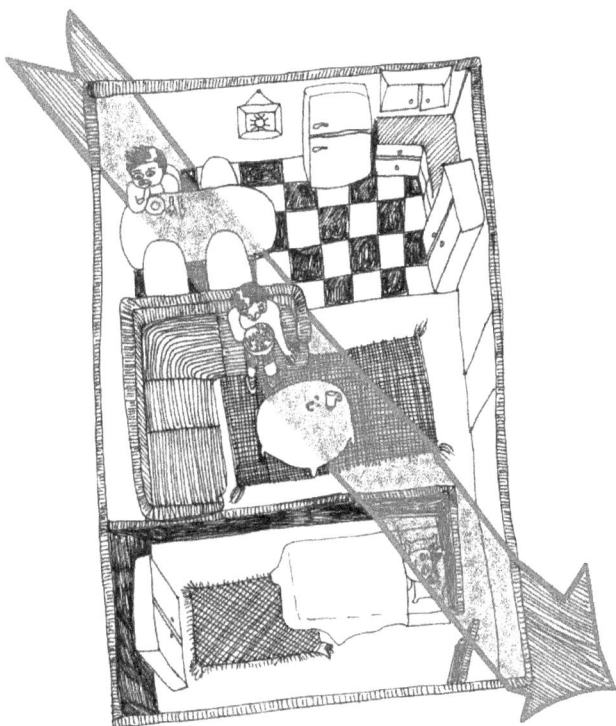

When my client had been there on her own, she slept on the other side of the bed, didn't sit at that end of the couch and never sat at that end of the dining table, in fact I think it was added when he moved in.

Simply by moving the bed slightly, moving the couch a metre one way and the table to the other side of the room, they noticed a huge difference within days.

He was also feeling better and recovering from his cold. His head was clearer; he was sleeping better and was not waking up angry and irritable. Their relationship improved all round.

Could moving the furniture really have made such a difference?

What if it was that easy?

HEART ISSUES

I had the chance to visit a house where the owner had been diagnosed with major heart issues as a result of blockages and wanted me to check her home.

On entering the house I started dowsing for Geopathic Stress that could be affecting anyone who lived in the home. I had never been in this house before and as always, I started from the front door and asked that no one tell me anything. i.e. who sleeps in which room or what issues they may have!

I always go into the house or building knowing nothing, so I am not being influenced in any way.

Once the dowsing is finished I will tell you what I find and discuss options to remedy the situation. Initially I picked up two lines downstairs crossing and causing a 'knot'. (This is where two lines cross each other so the energy intensifies) This knot was in the formal lounge; an area that didn't appear to get a lot of use, so I felt this would not be too much of a problem.

I then discovered another line crossing the dining table. While they had a house full of people that afternoon, I didn't feel this was a problem either as the table was large enough, and the family could fit around it without sitting in this noxious seat, and the table could be moved to avoid it.

Either way I hadn't found this to be too much of a problem at this point and typically you would only spend an hour at a time at the dining table.

On going upstairs, I detected the same lines I had picked up downstairs, however this was a whole different story. The two lines that had crossed in the formal lounge downstairs were in fact crossing on the owner's bed and you guessed it, directly affecting her heart area.

Naturally I recommended they move the bed immediately as it turned out they had slept in that position since moving into the house a decade earlier.

This noxious energy had been slowly aggravating her in exactly the same position every night, night after night, year after year for over 10 years!

What if it was that easy?

To just move their bed!

Well about 6 weeks later, she called to tell me that she had had her first check since the initial gruesome discovery. The healing process had actually improved far more than the Doctors had expected.

Mmmmmmm …..How come?

Was it the result of her moving off the noxious energy spot in her bedroom, and her body had the chance to start to heal itself!

Was the location of the bed the issue?

What if it was that easy?

AUTO IMMUNE DISEASE

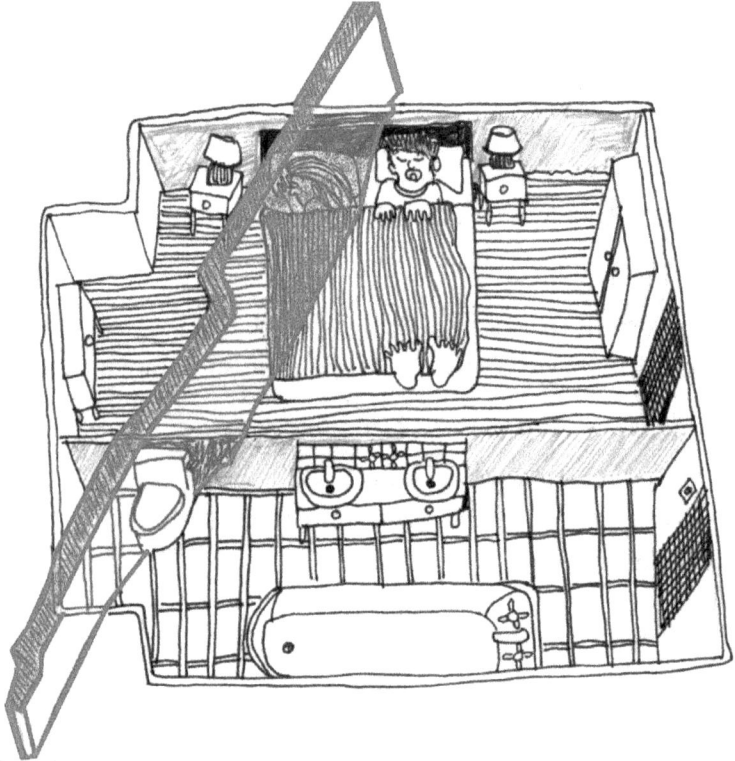

Another case is that of a beautiful lady I know who has a rare autoimmune disease that has plagued her body for many years. Even though I had suggested in the past that I felt she was a victim of GS, because all her symptoms were 'A-Typical' of someone who is suffering from this noxious earth energy called

Geopathic Stress.

- ✓ She got sick shortly after moving into the house,

- ✓ She got better when away on holiday or away from their house for any length of time.

Even though they had moved the bed years earlier as suggested, it was not until I had the chance to physically dowse the property on site recently that I was able to correctly detect where these Noxious Earth Energies were entering their home.

I found a line in the spare room before I entered the master bedroom and as I had never been in this house before, had no idea of the layout of the room before I opened the next door.

I found that the same line that ran through an area in the spare room but not really affecting any sleeping position, it did however affect the whole left side of the master bed in the main bedroom.

They told me that the bed was previously at 45deg to where it is now situated and this meant that the line ran directly across the bed. Which is where she would have slept, when she first got sick.

Now it ran from the base to the head of the bed on her side.

Being there, and showing her exactly where these lines were and how strong they were through the use of my dowsing rods, finally my beautiful friend recognized what I was talking about, when she saw the dowsing rods move, directly where she lay.

She had previously had professionals from around the world

pass their expert opinions, and recommending drug after drug be pumped into her body to help her, all seemingly just maintaining her life, but not improving it.

It has been only a short time since they have been sleeping completely in this new 'safe' position in their home and already they have both been noticing how much better they are feeling, and sleeping with more energy, a good nights sleep, has a flow through effect.

Previously they would be so tired that they would stay in bed until ten or eleven o'clock in the morning, sometimes even noon as they had no energy to get out of bed. Of course all this extra time they were spending in bed was actually making them worse.

After only a few weeks sleeping in this 'safe' GS free position they are up early each morning with renewed energy for the day! You can only imagine how different things could have been if 15 years ago, if I had the opportunity to physically 'show' them how serious this noxious earth energy is.

How many other people are in similar BBP positions? (Bad Bed Positions)

There are some more case studies later in the book.

What if it was that easy?

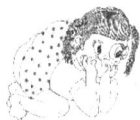

3 CHAPTER THREE

WHO ELSE IS AFFECTED?
ANIMALS AND PLANTS?

Who and what else indeed?

If we can be affected and of course babies and children seem to be even more sensitive than we as adults are, then who or what else are affected?

Have you been out driving and noticed rows of trees where one or two just aren't growing as fast as the rest.

Is Geopathic Stress affecting these?

I was trying to grow some vegetables in my garden, one side of the garden was amazing, and the other side just didn't seem to grow as well, even though they were the same plants and I used the same fertilizer.

Were these plants being affected by Geopathic stress or just dud plants and trees?

Highly likely I'd say!

My neighbor was growing a cute little boxed hedge and bought all the trees at the same time and they were all exactly the same.

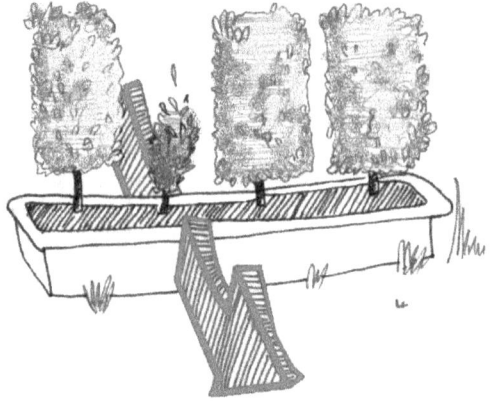

All were planted with the same love and passion, with the same soil, fertilizer, etc. But for some reason two trees directly opposite each other are just stunted. We all thought it was one of the neighborhood kids pouring something on them. Or was it a local dog that we had noticed, possibly urinating on them?

Is it possible that Geopathic Stress may affect them?

Yes it is very likely!

What about when I tried to plant some mint and parsley together in the same garden?

The mint grew really well, but the parsley didn't!

Well there is a good explanation for that, mint is attracted to the 'energy' created by Geopathic Stress and parsley is not. So if the area is affected in any way, one plant will do well and the other won't!

Just the same as Roses, Celery, Onions, Sunflowers, Aster, Azalea, Begonia, Geranium, Carnation, Primrose, Violet, Grape vines, Lilies and Cacti AVOID the negative energy caused by GS.

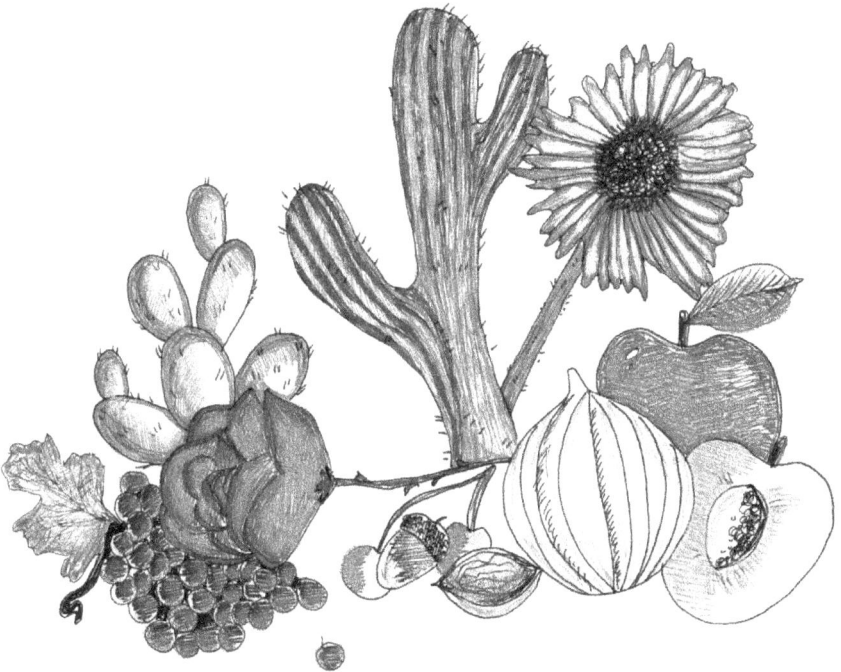

Also shrubs like Blackberry, Honeysuckle, Lilac, Blackcurrant, Buckthorn, Gooseberry and Hawthorn are in this bunch that do not like this energy.

Delicate trees like Apples, Pear, any nut bearing trees, Pecan, Walnuts, Macadamia etc. or even Ash, Beech, Willow, Oak, Pine, Apricot, Cherry, Lime, Sycamore, Larch, Poplar, Alder, Maple, Chestnut, Plum and Peach trees also DO NOT like the energy associated with Geopathic stress.

Just as we do not like this energy, neither do cows, sheep, pigs, horses, dogs, chickens, ducks pheasants, foxes, rabbits, mice, guinea-pigs, deer, badgers, storks, pigeons, birds, goats, and fish also do not like this energy.

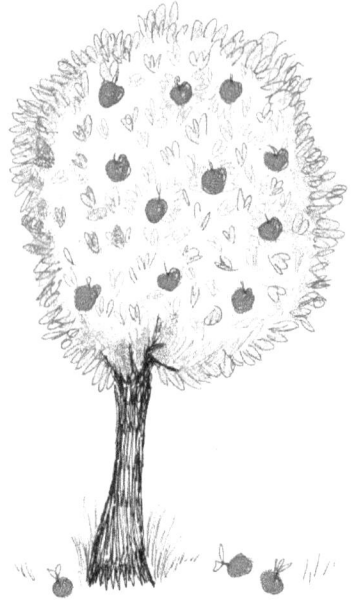

There are case studies that show where cows or horses that have been stabled in certain positions affected by GS are severely affected and have recurring injuries, or even worse.

Cows have been known to avoid an area in a milking shed where these energies are present.

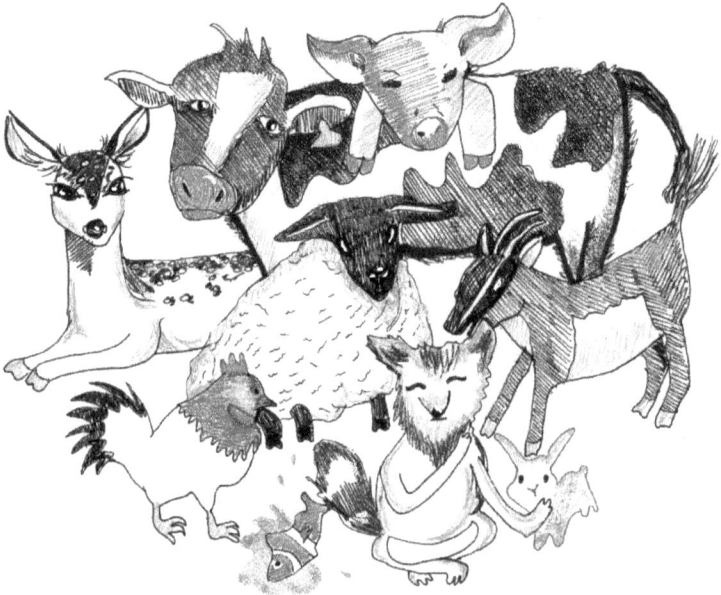

But on the opposite side of the coin, you know the 'Yin and Yang' side, some things like the energies.

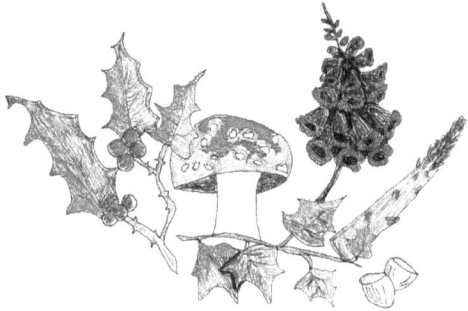

Something's have to LIKE this energy. Otherwise life would be unbalanced!

Although it is not necessarily the 'negative' energy they like, more like the heat and frequency that attracts them.

Some plants, for example that are drawn to the Noxious Earth Energy (GS) are Medicinal Herbs including verbena, marjoram, oregano, herb of grace, fenugreek, thistle, coltsfoot, mugwort, butterbur, nux vomica, foxglove, hemlock, bracken and nettles, Ivy, hazelnut, elderberry mistletoe, sea buckthorn, holly, belladonna, frankincense, juniper, cypress trees like it also Mushrooms, Asparagus and all weeds.

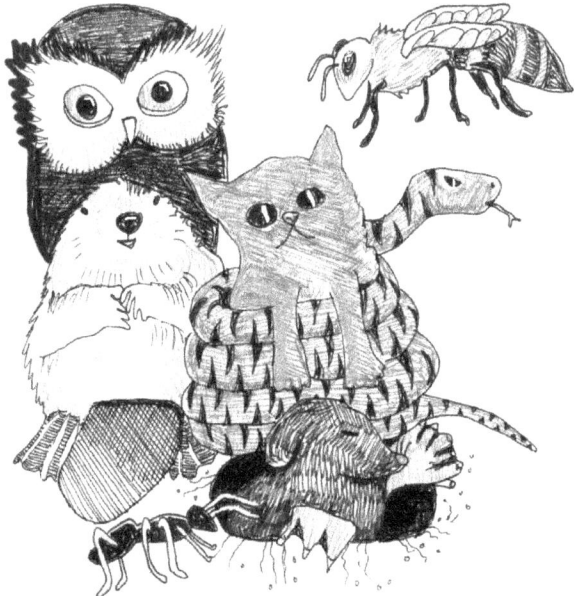

The animals that are drawn to this energy are

Cats, termites, ants, hornets, bees, wasp, owls, snakes,

Mosquitoes, moles,

Turtles, beavers and cockroaches and most other insects.

Have you been out walking and noticed trees that are twisted and others that are not?

I was playing golf recently and noticed a very distorted little forest with trunks that were all twisted from the bottom, yet the forest next to it the trees were tall and straight.

I bought it to my friend's attention that was with me and she made the comment that this was a coastal area and was it because of the sea winds.

I would say that could be the case if they were all leaning in the direction of the prevailing wind, but they weren't, they were just all twisted and almost looked in pain.

Many were actually pointing toward the prevailing winds, which I would think would be quiet unusual, as this was a fairly windy location.

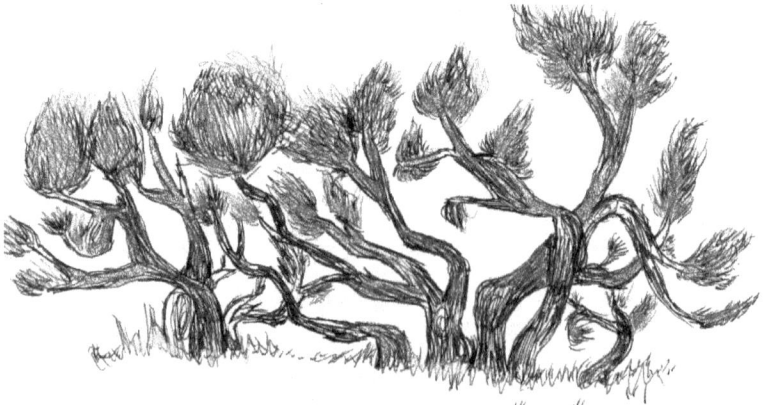

If I were to describe it, I would say they all were severely diseased.

Have you noticed trees like this?

Have you noticed cracks in the sidewalk, right beside distorted or diseased looking trees?

Have you noticed ants close to these areas?

Maybe you didn't know but you were noticing the effects of possible Geopathic stress.

So if it can affect trees, plants, and animals this clearly, then it makes it easier to see how we are affected. If this energy can affect a delicate plant then of course it can affect us.

The biggest problem we have is it seems too easy!

Especially if you have been brought up and have never been told about it before. Surely if it is this easy, you would have heard about it before right?

Is it really as simple as to just 'move off it'!

Also...Caged Animals and what happens to them?

Wow, now there is a huge subject that could fill a book all on its own. But here is the 'readers digest' version. If you have animals, whether they are chickens, pigs, horses or any other animal, and they are being restrained in a small area, that they can't naturally move away from the irritation of GS, what do you think it will do to them?

If they are horses and they are being 'stabled', it could cause injury!

Chickens won't lay or if they do, are the eggs 100% ok to eat or are they diseased?

If you have animals in shelters and there is an aggressive one, is this the one in the GS irritated cage?

Remember as I mention earlier, some animals are drawn to the frequency created by GS. But some like us humans are not! This is also a good indicator if there is an issue.

If your cat loves sleeping on your bed, or favourite chair, even if the sun isn't present and you are not there, chances are they have found the GS zone.

Dogs on the other hand are like us; they will be irritated and will not like it.

They will get fidgety and want to move away. They use to call it the 'Dog Test' in the old days (Oh my gosh I am soooo old). Actually it is way before my time.

They would put the dog in the location they wanted to put the bedroom in their house, and unrestrained the dog would have to 'sit' in that location without moving. If it moved away quickly, chances are it was no good for you!

Did you know that the dogs that they use at the airports to detect 'illegally carried food', have to be put in cages and cannot be taken home with the trainers?

What if they are being 'zapped' by GS where they sleep?

Or any other 'animals' that are trained for 'work' or our amusement, like at a Zoo etc. It does make you wonder if this may affect their personality.

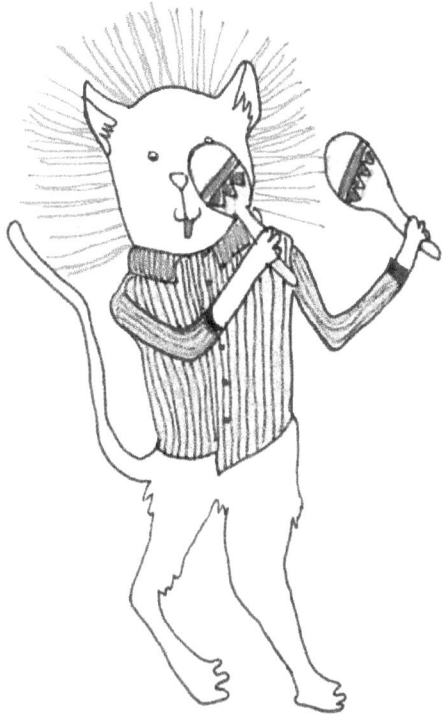

What if it was that easy?

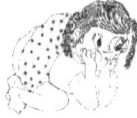

4 CHAPTER FOUR

IF GS IS ALWAYS THERE, THEN HOW CAN YOU BE SAFE?

It's like not being able to swim but being surrounded by water!

You would struggle and have no chance!

But if you have a life raft, then you'd be ok, right?

Of course you would, for a start, the main concern is really the places your spend time stationary! Unless your bed is in the water, you don't have a problem, as we can always move, slightly! This is your raft!

These energy lines aren't new!

Just because you haven't heard about them before, that doesn't mean they don't exist, or that you haven't many times in your life already been exposed to them.

They have been there since the beginning of time.

The Chinese knew about Geopathic stress over 4000 years ago and avoided building their homes on these geopathic lines, or Dragon Lines. Ancient civilizations around the world would never build their homes on these energy lines because they had the land they intended to build on dowsed first.

Some research shows up to 8000 years ago, cave drawings of them using rods to dowse for water.

So just to confirm, these Energy lines have been around for EVER!

Now to add to these Noxious Energy lines that were detected thousands of years ago, we have added our own pollution of EMF's and EMR's (Electro Magnetic Fields and Electrical Radiation) caused by Wi-Fi, mobile phones, telephone towers disguised as trees, electrics of all kind and much more, like excavation, mining, and all the other damage we do to the Earth.

Even dressed up as a tree, sadly these towers still emit huge radiation. Now where I live they don't even bother to disguise them, and they are everywhere.

As we are all cracking up when our mobile phones drop out, the Telco's are listening and they don't want to lose customers so what they do is put up more towers, and sadly now they don't even bother to disguise them.

Have a look around on the top of buildings when you are next out driving or walking or even just out in the open you will notice towers everywhere!

Therefore more radiation as the towers have to overlap so they don't risk you dropping out during your phone call, as this would risk them losing you as a customer.

Ok, so this is not going to go away! How do we protect ourselves without going into a state of depression and

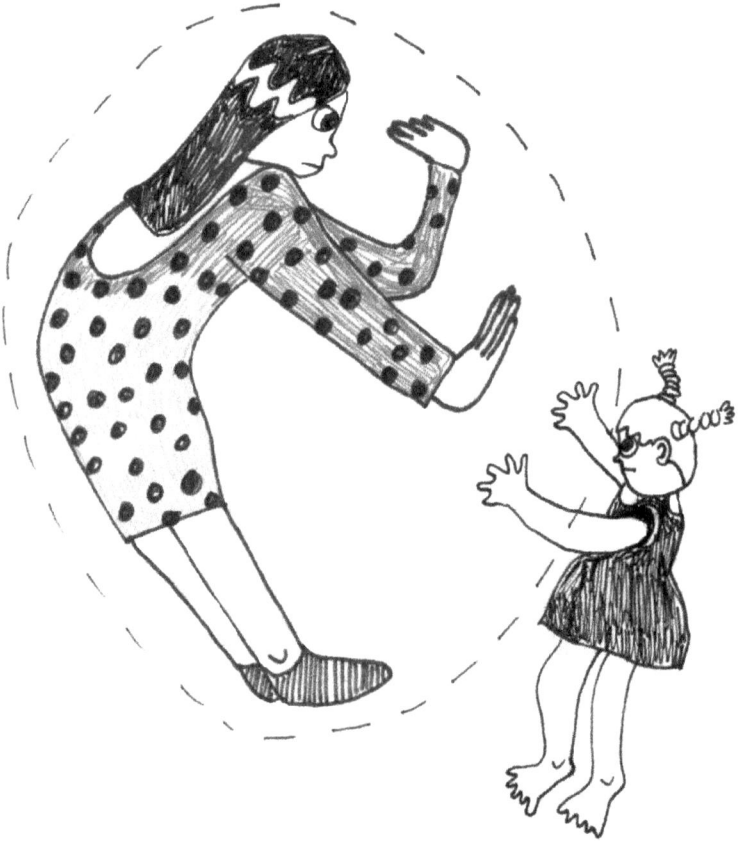

wrapping ourselves up in a glass bubble to hide from this?

Well that is not going to make for a very fun life, is it!

Being constantly wrapped in a bubble.

We still have to live our lives and that would not be 'living', well not how I want to live anyway.

What you do need to do is help make sure your 'immune' system is strong, full stop?

✓ Eat healthily,

✓ Exercise,

✓ Keep Stress levels at a manageable level,

✓ Laugh,

✓ Love,

And make sure you have your own personal crystal dome around yourself, but this must come from within.

Your Immune system is your crystal dome.

To keep your 'Immune' system strong, make sure that where you are spending the most time stationary i.e. bed, favourite chair, office desk etc. is clear from Geopathic stress and any Noxious Earth Energy.

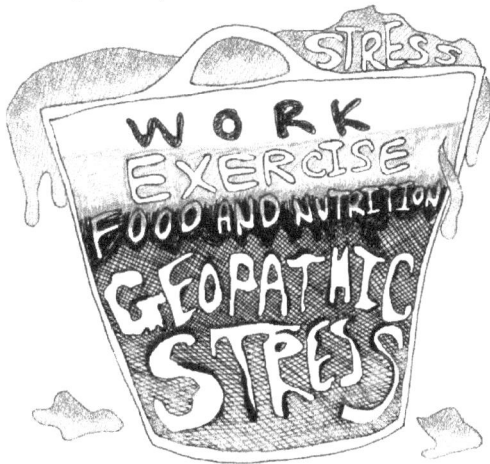

This is your own 'special secret weapon!

Keep your Immune system strong!

Easier said than done especially with all the invisible thin GS lines that bombard us every day, and I'm not talking about just GS this time.

What about the usual everyday stress or doozy 'out of the ordinary' stress, including internal and external we put ourselves through or all the radiation from cellphones, Wi-Fi, dirty electricity. etc. etc.! Your bucket will flow over if filled with all that.

WOW, what can we do when we are surrounded?

Firstly don't panic because that isn't going to help anyone, especially you..

Your bucket is far less likely to overflow without all that Geopathic Stress in it.

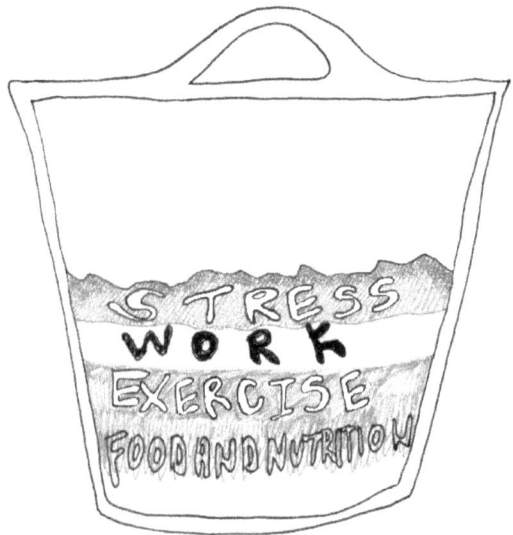

But on top of that, the best way to help make this happen is when we spend time in bed, which on average humans sleep for approximately 1/3 of our lives, between 6-9 hours a day.

✓ Be clear and safe!

✓ **Remember the 'Secret is Clear Energy'!**

Now can you understand why it is so important to keep your immune systems strong!

Empty your bucket of Geopathic Stress! So make sure that your bed is in a Geopathically stress free safe zone! i.e. No geopathic stress, reduced EMF's and EMR's. These are very hard to completely eradicate unless you want to live in Whip-Whop miles from everywhere with absolutely no electricity and certainly no Wi-Fi or neighbour's that may have them!

This is how to keep your Immune system strong.

I have found with all my customers who believed they were being affected by EMF's or EMR's were first being irritated by GS.

Of course as I already mentioned you have to eat a healthy well balanced diet with fresh fruits and vegetables, good proteins, exercise regularly and keep your stress levels low.

As my darling Grandmother use to always say "Everything in moderation" and she lived to the ripe ole age of 101.

Now most importantly 'BE AWARE!

Get your 'gut' tuned in, so you can FEEL this energy, and move off it.

By 'gut', I mean INTUITION!

(More on that later in the book)

If you move into a new house, whether you purchase it or are just renting, it is irrelevant, you are still 'living' in that space so you MUST make sure it is safe for you and your family.

Don't trust that just because you have a nice new house that it is completely 'safe and healthy'! It could be brand new or have been recently re decorated with all new materials so how can there be an issue, right!

Did you test the land before you built or bought?

It could be even worse if you have lived in a house for a long period of time. Check yourself?

- ✓ Do a health check on yourself!

- ✓ Do a health check on your House!

- ✓ Has your health deteriorated since you moved in?

- ✓ Were you healthy before you moved in?

- ✓ How are you feeling now, compared with then?

- ✓ Are you blaming your age for your bad health?

- ✓ Could it possibly be a location-based illness?

- ✓ Do you blame it or say it's 'hereditary'?

Are the illnesses or conditions that plague a family due to the fact they live in the same house and could have been irritated by the same noxious energy?

Could it really be that easy?

What if your bed was causing your health problems?

And that doesn't mean you have to run out and buy a new bed, *just move it!*

What if my bed can't be moved?

Are you then stuck with being affected with 'Negative Noxious Earth Energy'?

Thank goodness no!

There is always an option! The first thing I would always recommend is to find a clear space away from this energy.

If the energy has been so strong that it can come from deep under the earth, then moving away from it will be the best and safest option.

But first you need to know where these energy lines are?

HOW ARE YOU GOING TO SEE THEM?

Do they have a colour or can you feel them?

Well yes and no! Some people can see them as colours, but the rest of us who dowse can 'feel' them, or sense them.

If you can't feel them yourself, you can contact a 'dowser' or 'geomancer' to come to your home or business to detect these for you. You will have felt them, as a hot or cold feeling walking into a room or a chill down your spine, or a tingling.

We've all felt that at times right?

Some dowsers like myself, can even Distance Dowse anywhere around the world, but I'll tell you more about that later. Check out chapter eight for more information.

If you have managed to live your life until now and never known about GS, why do you need to know about it now, right?

My parents didn't know about it? They're still alive!

The illnesses that some people have in their lives were just 'in the family'!

They are hereditary aren't they?

What if the family home was causing their illnesses? Rather than 'something' that may be genetic and passed down!

What if their bedroom had Geopathic Stress running through it and the heart attack that your Father, Grandfather, Uncle, or Friend had was not passed down from generation to generation, but was where they had put their body night after night?

Did the same GS line ran through the bedrooms on that side of the house and therefore affect all the rooms? Often the bedrooms may be in a line on one side of the house, I just had this recently and each bedroom had GS crossing the beds. If the plan had been reversed it would have crossed the kitchen and bathrooms and not been such an issue.

What if the breast cancer that your Mother, Aunt, Sister, Grandmother or friend had was also aggravated by where they chose to sleep?

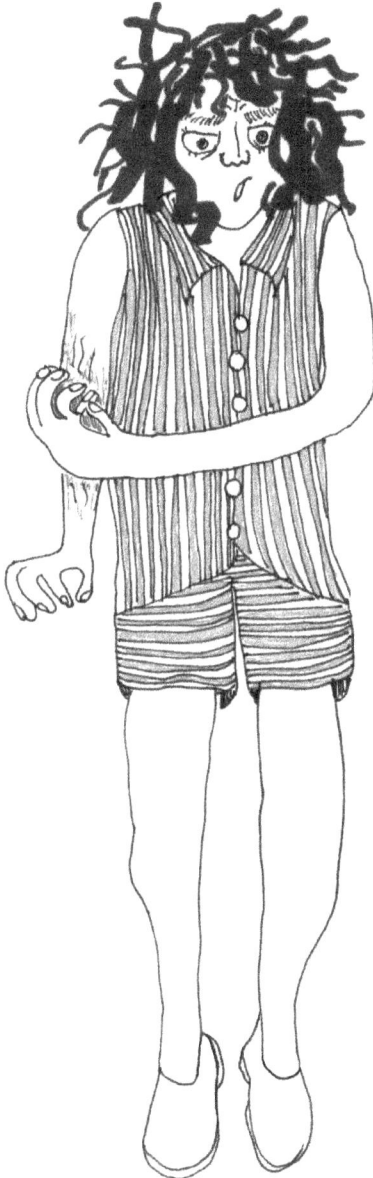

Or if you are a man, is the prostate issue you are experiencing being blamed on the lineage passed down from your Dad or Grandfather?

What if the bed wetting that you suffered as a child was caused by the way your bedroom was laid out. And those horrific nightmares that plagued your childhood were from your cozy little bed, or the location of it?

Especially as a teenager you are even more susceptible as you have many hormones going crazy in your body and are even more sensitive to GS.

What if the acne you just can't get rid of as a teenager is only affecting

67

you and not your sibling, yet you are eating the same food and living the same lifestyle. Except you are sleeping in a different bed?

Could it be that easy?

What if the learning difficulties you or someone you know, had at school was where you were sleeping and/or were in the classroom you sat or even did your homework at home?

What if asthma, psoriasis and eczema and other skin conditions you have experienced in your life weren't necessarily passed down from your parents or a genetic issue, but rather are a 'location' issue?

You could be blaming the food you are eating and have tried every eating regime to help curb the terrible skin problems, or have to use all the horrible steroid creams to help, but every night you go and sleep in the same place?

What if the unsettled baby that doesn't sleep night after night

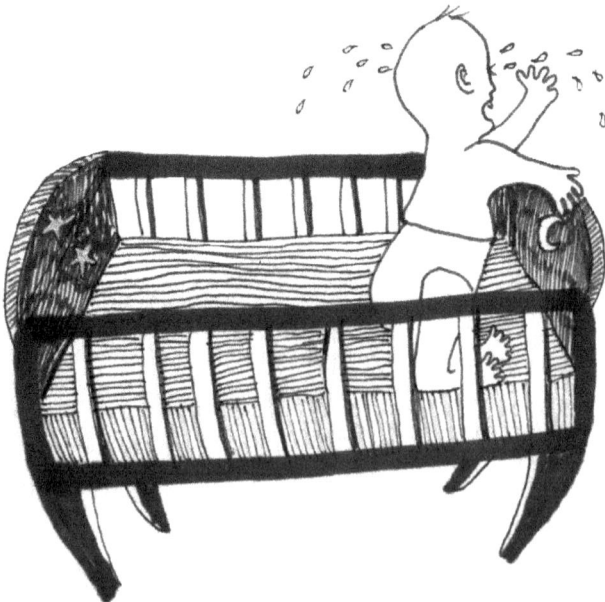

and is driving you crazy and exhausting you, is from where you decided to put their bassinet or cot?

Babies and children are sensitive and are not being told by society that this 'invisible energy' is not affecting them. If they don't feel well they are going to let you know very quickly. I wish I knew about this when I had my babies, as when I look back now there is a definite link to the locations I placed them.

I actually dowsed the plan of the house we owned many years ago, when my children were babies. My daughter nearly died as a young baby. She was asleep in a bassinet beside our bed when she was round three months old. I luckily happened to still be up doing some sewing and my husband was sound asleep in our bed next to her bassinet.

I heard an unusual noise and ran in to find her 'blue' and not breathing. We jolted her little body and luckily she started breathing. She was rushed to hospital and had a series of tests. They could not find any reason she had stopped breathing but we could have lost her if I hadn't heard that noise.

Twenty nine years later, she is a blessing and well and truly alive. But I was thinking about this near tragedy the other day and decided to 'Distance Dowse' our old house, using Google maps.

I found a 'knot' exactly where I had placed her bassinet in our room, and also in her bedroom when she transferred into a cot on the other side of the house was a Geopathic Stress line of energy crossing directly through her room. In this bedroom it was a constant 'issue' to get her to bed. She would constantly cry, and always ended up at the wrong end of the cot. I could never put her down to sleep in her cot during the day and would just leave her in her pram in the lounge as she slept really well in that. Now I know it was obviously in a 'GS clear' space from the plan I dowsed.

The other thing I remembered recently was in the same house prior to when I had my daughter and she had suffered the attack mentioned, I had suffered an 'Ectopic Pregnancy'!

This is where you get pregnant and the embryo implants somewhere outside the uterus. It was a very serious situation and sadly I ended up in intensive-care for 3 days. But luckily even with only one tube I managed to get pregnant later. However it does make me wonder if the location where my bed was and if GS had anything to do with the malfunction of my system to let the embryo form in the fallopian tube. Was the GS irritation too strong?

If only I had known then about Geopathic Stress. I would have had my house 'dowsed' for GS and other Noxious Energies before we bought the house and certainly before I brought my baby home to live in it. My son's bedroom was clear of GS. He never had an issue sleeping at night.

I can hear myself now saying "I wonder why she doesn't sleep like her brother"!

How many other parents are out there saying exactly the same thing?

Sadly when we moved to the next house (where we lived for nearly 15 years) the GS was also affecting her new bedroom.

And for some reason my son's bedroom was again clear of GS. It just goes to show that our health may be a result of pot-luck!

Pot-Luck which bedroom we choose or is chosen for us!

What if the cot death (SIDS) that affected your family or someone you know, wasn't the mystery you all thought it was?

What if it was where they unknowingly placed the bassinet or cot in the house? What if the vibration or frequency caused by GS was too strong for the new baby or unborn baby? Or even you were affected when you were pregnant and then placed the cot in an area that was also affected, the baby would be irritated easily. What's more they will let you know, so if your baby doesn't sleep and they are not hungry or wet, check the location of where they are sleeping.

What if the injury you received outside your home, i.e. falling over and breaking a limb or spraining an ankle, or an injury that is not responding to treatment is being caused by where you are sleeping. Or that part of your body has been weakened and aggravated every time you go to bed.

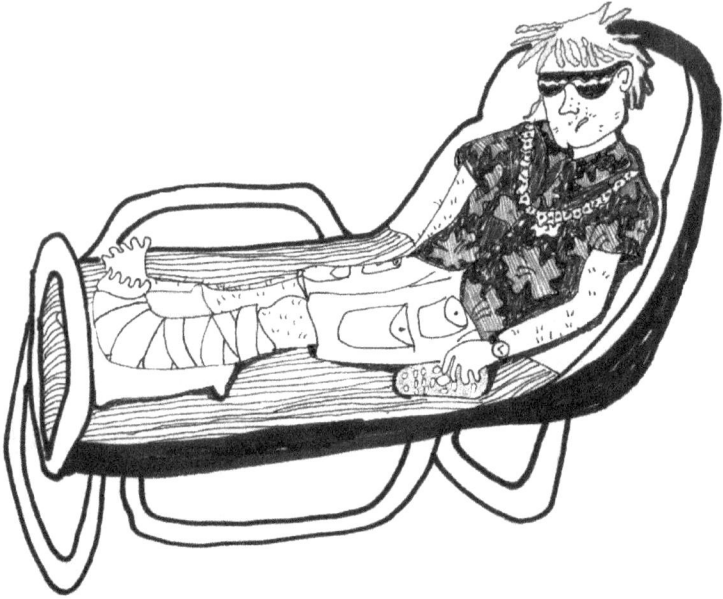

And every night when you come home to rest and recuperate is actually causing you more harm than good!

One step forward and two steps back! If you are sleeping in a GS clear zone, there is no question it will help speed up the usual recovery time. I have had exactly this situation with one of my clients recently.

What if that marriage breakup that split your family up, wasn't the fact that you two just couldn't stand the sight of each other anymore, but was caused by where you were both sleeping?

The irritation you were experiencing while you were asleep, was rubbing on both of you to the point where you wanted to kill each other and sadly the relationship broke up.

Did you notice that the people that used to live in the house where you now live also had a split marriage?

Did you even ask why they were selling?

In fact, the last three owners previous to you, also had marriage break ups?

Who cares right, as that is why we got the house cheap! They needed to get out of there fast.

What if it was that easy?

What if the fighting siblings in your family that appear to never be at peace and are always at each other's throats, is caused by which beds they chose to sleep in or were put in by the parents?

What if the one child that was so different to other children you had also had learning difficulties, ADHD, and struggles with anti-social behavior were they being affected by the bed they slept in?

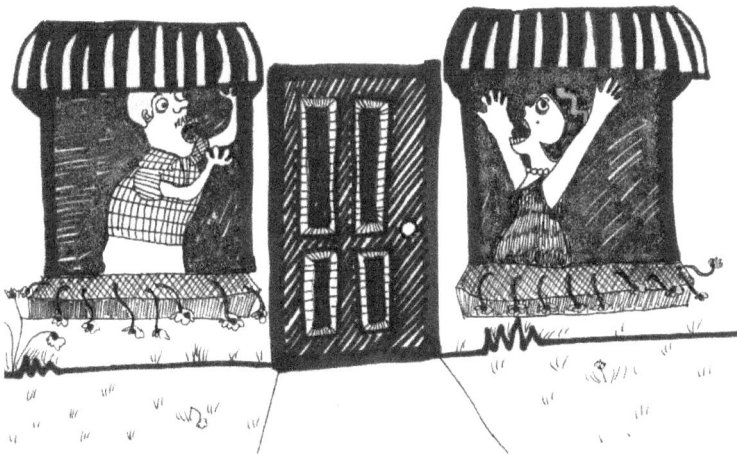

Are they like that because of where they were sleeping?

Is it a 'location illness'?

Could it be that easy?

What if your weight issues, either not being able to lose weight or put on weight and the lack of appetite in the mornings was caused by where you put your head at night?

What if that loss of sex drive you and your partner are experiencing is because of where you put your bed when you moved into your home?

Not because you ate too much and drank too much, or maybe you just don't like each other anymore?

But what if it's not?

What if that high blood pressure and all those drugs you are taking to help lower it, are actually not working because of where you are working all day at your desk, and in fact this is actually causing it.

Or those migraines that you constantly have are in fact caused by that position you are sitting at work?

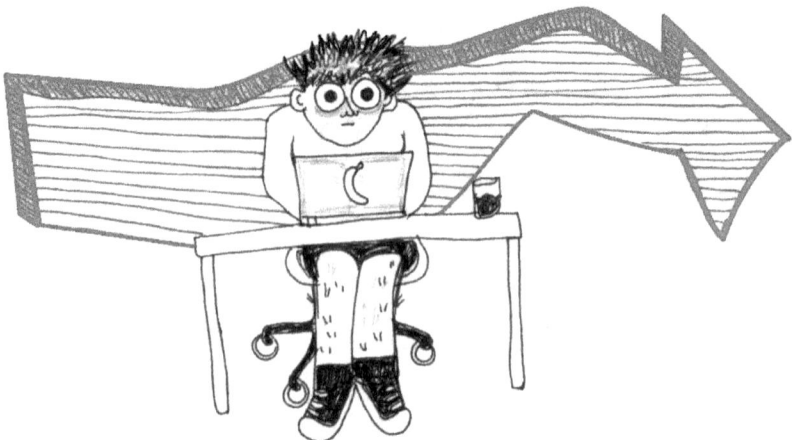

What if those anxiety attacks you have been experiencing are actually from the bed you chose to sleep in.

And I don't mean the type of bed, or the softness or how hard it is? I mean 'where' it is!

What if the diarrhea, constipation, cramping and bloating that you have, is not caused by the food you thought was affecting you, but rather the location you were spending time sleeping, or sitting was affecting your digestive and intestinal system and therefore affecting you with those symptoms?

Just remember where you sit at work or in the office, you are upright therefore if there is GS running through that location, even MORE of your body could be affected than in your bed.

Many people unfortunately spend longer at work than bed. If you are not loving your job and constantly get sick or irritated easily, get back-ache, headaches or migraines, then you need to check for GS in your office.

Don't forget we are also adding electromagnetic radiation in every office.

Everyone has a cellphone if not two, Wi-Fi, printers, (usually all talking to each other through Wi-Fi), plus many other electrical products, laptops, computers, tablets, not counting all the dirty electricity from wiring etc. etc. etc..

But if we start from the ground (meaning Earth Energies first) and eliminate or identify where they are, then 'electrical and other magnetic fields' or as it's known now 'Technostress' are easier to see and identify.

More on that later.

What if the Crohns or Celiac (Coeliac) disease and/or Chronic Fatigue that has taken over your body and completely affecting your life, was indeed caused by the location of your bed?

- ✓ Where does it end?

- ✓ What have you just accepted as a normal part of aging and life?

- ✓ Are any of these in fact fixable by you?

- ✓ Why hasn't anyone ever told you this?

- ✓ Why did you not know this before?

- ✓ What if it was that easy?

You cannot be blamed for 'not knowing'.

But now it's time to 'know'!

Now it's time to 'learn'!

For hundreds of years this knowledge was kept a secret, as they didn't want everyone to know. They knew how powerful it was!

Maybe in the hands of the wrong people it could change the world?

Don't you have the right to make that choice for yourself?

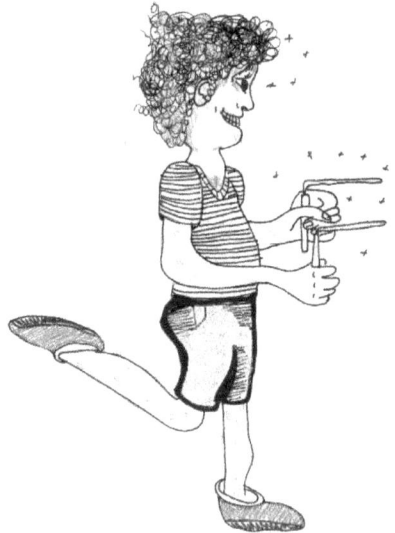

If you have the chance to help 'Heal your Home or Office', therefore giving yourself, your family or staff and work colleagues the best possible grounding for a healthy life, don't you deserve that chance?

Damn right you do!

And this is where it starts.

Is it that easy?

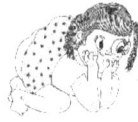

5 CHAPTER FIVE
WHY DID'T YOU KNOW ABOUT THIS BEFORE?

If this weird thing is as serious as the indications mentioned, why haven't you heard about Geopathic Stress and Noxious Earth Energy before?

How could something so simple be so serious, and be hidden under the bed, or under my desk or chair at work?

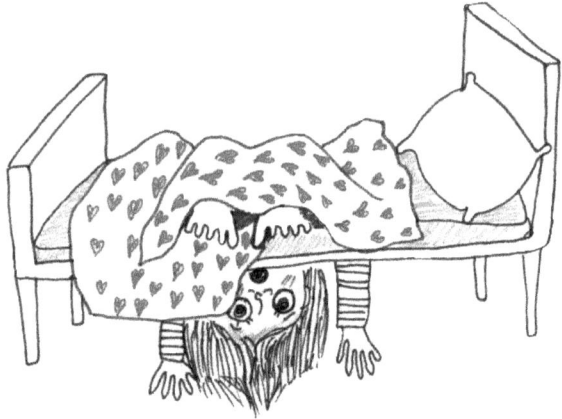

This should be shouted from the rooftops and be part of everyone's 'knowledge', so it is something we automatically would check when moving into a home, apartment, flat, office, building, farm, tree house etc.

Agreed?

If you have a 'Building Biology/Geomancy' check done before you move into a new house/flat/apartment and place your bed, children's beds, lounge, home office, etc. in safe (GS free zones) you will be aware where these lines are so you can avoid them and be protected in the future. From Geopathic Stress anyway.

At least then, you know you are providing you and your family's 'system' the best chance to live a fulfilled life free from GS.

If down the track, symptoms happen to occur again you can re-check your Geomancy plan so that all the places you or your family are spending time are still safe, then you can get on with your lives and know that any other traditional treatments you choose won't be slowed down or their effects reduced by GS.

At least you will know that the treatments you are paying for have all the opportunity to work and are not likely to be undermined by this invisible Noxious Earth energy.

Sometimes, if we have droughts, floods, earthquakes or other 'acts of god' some of these energy lines can move slightly so it is good to check in with it periodically.

It is such a simple solution for such a complex problem.

So then why didn't you know about this before?

Was it because the 'dowsers' used to be only the Ordained Priest and it was like a secret society? They knew the power of these energy lines and didn't want the 'great unwashed' to know about them.

They also knew where they were and would use these strong powerful lines and knots to their advantage.

All the churches and temples around the world are placed very carefully over these lines so the pulpit where the priest would command his sermons was on one of these powerful 'knots'.

Hey.. But didn't you say that spending too much time on these lines can affect your health?

Yes you are right. But for short periods of time they are 'charging' them with energy and this would provide the priest a strength and the power he needed to deliver a powerful sermon.

If you weren't an ordained priest, people who practiced geomancy were known as 'water witches' and were burnt at the stake as people didn't understand their power, ability and gift to detect these energies.

I believe at least 50-70% of people can dowse and detect these energies and of course they can affect 100% of us.

Unfortunately many the fathers, grandfathers, mothers and grandmothers that knew of the gift and knowledge of dowsing or divining died in wars and did not have the chance to pass on their knowledge?

Why has this knowledge disappeared?

Is it because we weren't surrounded by technology like we are now that can cloud our judgment? We have turned off our intuition.

Was it because we had more room and space to build our homes and we 'felt' where was the right place to put them?

Were our rooms larger and we had more space to move things around?

Were we more active and not spending as much time stationary?

Some cultures used things like termite nests or dogs to test the location. If the termites stayed there, then they knew that was not a good place for them to put their bedroom.

But if the dog stayed there un-restrained, then this would be a good place.

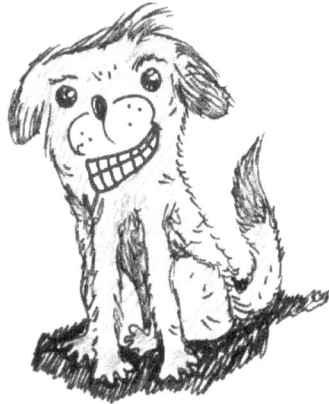

In some cultures they would watch and take note where the cattle slept. After a year when they killed the beast for food they would check the liver and if it was clear they knew that was a good place for them to build their home.

When we didn't have technology like we do today, we 'did' things outside. We moved around a lot and were never stationary, unless we were asleep.

I remember when I was younger we never stayed inside. We used every opportunity to get out of the house otherwise you had to do the dishes…no dishwashers then! Oh my gosh, I'm so old, ha-ha!

Is it because we are now more space poor and have to build our homes on top of each other and live in apartment blocks, or on smaller sections with smaller rooms so we have less chance of creating that 'clear' space?

Or is it because we all have mobile phones and Wi-Fi in our homes and we are not only being affected by the Wi-Fi and electronics in our homes? Our neighbour's are also so close we are picking up disturbances with their Wi-Fi as well? I'm not sure about you but everyone in my family has a mobile phone.

How many people in your family have a mobile phone?

In your office how many?

Are we wiring up our homes for operating this and that and also for future needs? Things like cabling for speakers, lights, or that sound system and don't forget the additional ones we may need one day! Everything is getting so automated, and more things are now run wireless. If

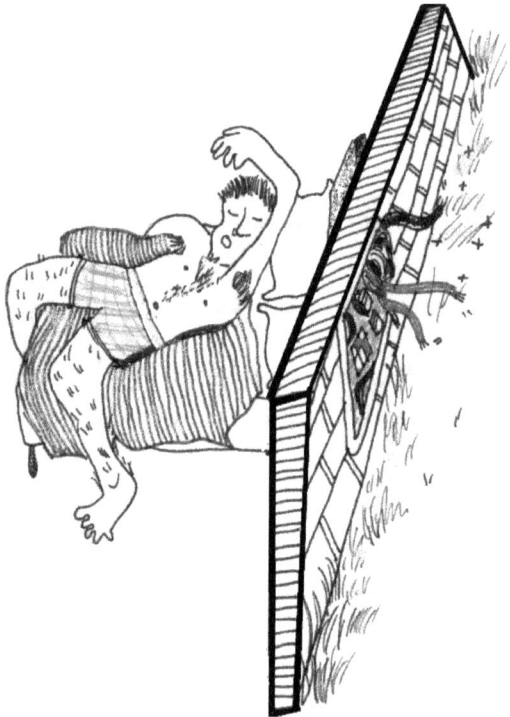

it's wireless, then there is a 'signal' somewhere.

Sadly all that cabling and wireless is great as it enables a speaker in every corner of your house, but it also carries electro-magnetic smog and dirty electricity.

I have a friend who was being affected by GS in his house, but also EMF's. He was diagnosed with bone-marrow leukemia and went through all the necessary chemo and other treatments and thankfully it pulled him through.

However after returning home luckily his wife was determined to have a building biology test done on their home and found that the wall in their bedroom directly behind his head had all the cabling for the entire house running through it.

So every night they went to bed and more than likely his side of the bed would have been affected by Geopathic Stress. All that Electro Magnetic Smog was zapping him directly on his head.

I am sure that if the power cables were visible instead of being hidden behind 10-12ml of plasterboard, there is no way he would have put his bed up against that wall each night.

How many other people are in exactly the same position?

Luckily he moved the position of his bed and many years later he is still alive and well. He has had a couple of slight relapses, and it has coincided with moving homes and new position he was sleeping in which also turned out to be affected by GS.

When you have been in a situation where your immune system has been compromised and you have been affected by Cancer,

MS, Chronic Fatigue, Heart Attacks/Diseases, or any other serious illnesses, it is important to make sure that your bed is as safe and healthy as possible.

It is the time when we are stationary in our beds that we need our body to be healing and rejuvenating to the best of its ability. With 6-9 hours lying still in one place it is the perfect chance to recharge the system.

I say 'bed' as it's where most people spend the most time stationary. As I mentioned many people spend extended time in their offices that are badly affected by GS in fact some up to 10-12 hours a day sitting in the same position, so this space is just as important to check to ensure it's just as safe, and to be fair even safer.

At work, many are also surrounded by EMF's (computers, mobile phones, Wi-Fi and everything else in between) as well. If you work in an industrial area chances are all the other buildings around you have lots going on as well.

You don't typically have a lot of electronics in your bedroom, and if you do – get rid of them!

That includes electric blankets and magnetic blankets as well. Buy a feather topper pad, and you will never need an electric blanket again.

Do not have radio alarm clocks especially digital ones beside your bed. If you saw the radiation that is emitted from them you wouldn't want them close to your head.

If you do have them put them on the other side of the room so you actually have to get out of bed to turn them off. That is what you are supposed to do, instead of hitting the 'snooze' button all the time. Just set it for the right time and get up.

Once you are clear of all this electromagnetic smog and no GS, you might find you don't need an alarm and just bounce out of bed.

Well here's hoping.

Also your mobile phones should be as far from your head as possible while you are sleeping. Charge them on the other side of the room as far away from your head and body as possible so you have to get up to turn off.

Every metre away from your head your phone is reducing the EMF and EMR (that's the electrical radiation) while you are sleeping.

Don't forget sleep deprivation is the worst torture so why would we allow something so critical to our survival continue in this day and age, when we don't need to!

If Geopathic Stress never shuts off and you are sleeping 6-9 hours a night and also working on a GS zone during the day up to 12 hours, then the stress hormones (cortisol) produces feelings of anxiety and helplessness. Oversensitivity to Geopathic Stress has been linked with severe depression because depressed people have a harder time adapting to the negative side affects of cortisol (stress hormone).

Excessive amounts of cortisol can cause sleep disturbances, loss of sex drive, and a general lack of interest in sex.

Now that's enough reason to move your bed isn't it?

Depression and anxiety may contribute to illness and this may cause people to be depressed or anxious.

Tense muscles can cause headaches and neck pain.

But if people eliminate Geopathic Stress from their lives they could have no further adverse health and emotional conditions, or certainly reduce them.

The trick is eliminating it, or at least identifying where it is, so you can move off it.

In short bursts elevated adrenalin is not damaging or dangerous. In fact, that is what it is designed to do.

But when sustained at high levels over a long period of time it can be very harmful.

Such long-term over-arousal and excessive flow of this hormone will eventually lead to physiological and psychological distress.

You do not want it to get to this level so best thing is to have a building biology test done on your home and/or work place, or learn to do it yourself!

More about that in Chapter Eight!

'RELOCATE DON'T MEDICATE'!

And that might mean only moving half a metre.

Before you take all those headache pills drink lots of water as hydration is so important to keep those headaches and migraines away, then make sure the places that give you those headaches are not Geopathically stressed!

Notice where you get those headaches?

Do you wake up with them?

Is it at your computer?

Is it on the couch or at the dining table?

What if it's a certain location?

Could it be that easy?

What if it was?

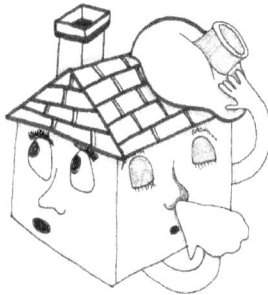

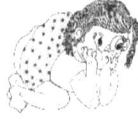

6 CHAPTER SIX
DIFFERENCE BETWEEN GEOMANCY &
FENG SHUI

Feng Shui (means wind and water)

For some reason it seems to have so many different pronunciations.

If you are from the UK, you pronounce it "Feng Shu'ee' and if you are from the US is sounds more like " Fung Sh'way'!

Either is correct and mean the same thing, just different accents!

It started with the ancient Chinese Masters that studied the earth patterns so they could decide the best places to put their homes and buildings.

They were described as Geomancy Masters, so that would indicate that there is a link between Geomancy and Feng Shui, if not the very base or heart of it.

As legend would have it, the ancient Chinese were very careful where they placed their burial sites. In this process they would dowse to identify where the most auspicious energy was so they could place their ancestors to rest and this would satisfy the spirits and ensure the ongoing protection and help needed for future lives.

Feng Shui is a beautiful powerful sensing of energy and is designed to maximize the potential in every situation to help the life force of the people who live or work in these spaces.

With the power of Feng Shui and Geomancy we have the gift to be able to identify and transform any place into a harmonious place, which is why these 'arts' are becoming more popular all over the world.

If the practitioner is qualified and has taken 'ego' out of the equation they have the ability to be able to harmoniously add healing to the energies in the home therefore add healing to the occupants.

Consider where in the world you live as Feng Shui originated in the Northern Hemisphere and the rules change if you live in the Southern hemisphere. So check where you are in the world.

Some say that Geomancy and Feng Shui are not the same, but in my belief they are one and the same, in fact Geomancy is really the science under Feng Shui. You cannot have one without the other.

As humans we are ultimately a mysterious lot and we are learning every second of every day more and more about what makes us tick. The deep mysteries that Geomancers have been trying to discover since the beginning of time.

If Feng Shui and Geomancy can help uncover some of these mysteries to make our lives as humans kinder, healthier, and create a more peaceful and happier race of people then this is indeed a wonderful time to be alive.

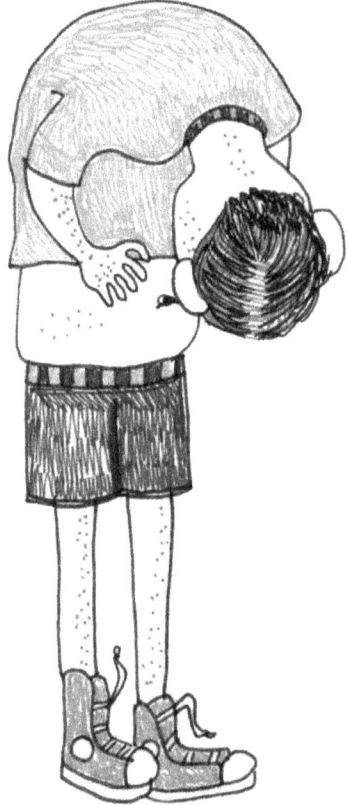

There is debate as to whether Feng Shui or Geomancy started in China or Europe but as yet no one seems to have that answer. All ancient cultures have some form of geomancy and divination and they have all used these arts adopting various techniques to help them to find water, and where to place their homes in safe 'clear' places, so they can have the healthiest lives for their communities.

They would listen to the land and they knew instinctively where it was good for them.

We have lost that art!

We have stopped listening!

There are too many other things to listen to so we get confused and don't know what to listen to any more so we shut down. Or we listen to the ones who have the biggest voices. They are usually the ones with the biggest budgets, and not necessarily the ones we should be listening to.

Why has cancer, heart disease and diabetes increased so much from a time when we lived and listened to the land?

We all donate so much every year to get the magic answers we need about these diseases, but maybe we just need to 'LISTEN' to our gut or follow our intuition? Of course there is no way I am suggesting that you don't listen to your Doctor or Health professional, I am simply saying you must also listen to your own inner wisdom. If someone says something to you and it doesn't feel right, get another opinion. It's your body and YOU are the only one that can HEAR it as well as you can.

I find it interesting the number of times that I've gone into someone's home who has had their place "fenged' (as it's sometimes referred) by a professional Feng Shui consultant, and when I move the furniture away from Geopathic Stress and into a new location that would go against the grain of a Feng Shui consultant, the whole room feels better. I regularly get calls from clients whose homes or offices I have dowsed, where I have only taken into consideration the Geopathic Stress and the health of people as a result of that, and have been amazed.

They come back to me and say the whole place feels better.

The other information I find really interesting is about Gypsies.

This came from the *Dulwich Health Society in the UK says that they (Gypsies) have very low incidence of heart disease and cancer. This is because they are continually on the move.

Queen Victoria had dowser find the best place for her holiday home, which is where 'Balmoral Castle' is located today.

She was eighty-one when she died. The Queen Mother was 101 when she died, and Queen Elizabeth II turns 90 this year. Just saying!

Maybe we should all get into the habit of changing sides of the bed more often. I know so many of my clients have a preferred 'side' and will only sleep on a certain side of the bed even when they go away on holiday. Change is so much fun, give it a try!

How many of you ALWAYS sleep on one particular side of the bed and NEVER change?

We are such creatures of habit and sometimes this can be to our detriment!

This in itself seems a good reason to moving occasionally, even if it's just to the other side of the bed.

What if it was that easy?

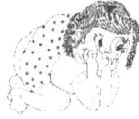

7 CHAPTER SEVEN
CASE STUDIES FROM ALLERGIES TO BEDWETTING & CANCER TO WEIGHT-GAIN

Listed below are a few of the diseases that have been linked to Geopathic Stress and a number have actual case studies associated with them.

Of course there are many other illnesses and diseases linked to GS that are not mentioned. What I do know, especially if your immune system or lack of immunity is causing the disease that is affecting you, then get it checked out to make sure GS isn't a factor.

Studies show that up to 85% of chronic illnesses are linked to GS.

ALLERGIES:

Allergies are getting more and more prevalent in today's society. Peanut allergies for example were never heard of when I went to school, so what's has happened in the last 20 years? Cell towers? Increased telecommunications, and everyone, I mean everyone has Wi-Fi and cellphones and sometimes more than one for work and personal use.

If you have a grown up family of four chances are there are 4 phones in the home. Even young children seem to have them nowadays.

I heard on the TV today, that there are more registered mobile phones in New Zealand than there are people. Wow! I guess this is indicative of many modern societies around the world.

Therefore we need more cell towers around to cope with them. Could this be causing the increased sensitivity to everyone? Are our immune systems getting so overloaded with EMF's (Electromagnetic Frequencies) that the cells in our bodies just throw their little hands up and go ENOUGH! (you need to imagine your cells have arms here) They say 'I can't cope', so something has gotta give.

Our skin is the largest and fastest growing organ in our body so it's likely that it is going to be the first to give way, when things get too tough.

Are we giving our precious skin the best chance?

Make sure it is getting the fresh air, water, healthy food and of course rest (i.e. GS free) that it needs to be the best looking living skin you can have.

ARTHRITIS:

I was diagnosed with 'chronic arthritis' nearly 20 years ago. It was so bad, that I had to have cortisone injections directly into my toe joints to relieve the pain even though I have a high pain tolerance. I would have regular podiatry appointments, and had special orthotics made (at great expense) for my feet to help with the pain. Rheumatologists confirmed with X-Rays that I indeed had Arthritis. However after moving my bed to a safe "GS free zone' the arthritis is today nowhere to be found.

I have no signs of it anymore, and yet I was told it was all 'doom and gloom' from the specialists at the time.

How many other people out there have also had diagnosis of something similar and maybe just need to relocate where they spend time stationary. i.e. move your bed! (But do make sure it is a 'GS clear space')

AGGRESSION & SUDDEN IRRITABILITY:

I have had many customers who have experienced first-hand aggression and certainly sudden irritability and often with their children. Blaming things like the Terrible Twos or "Oh they are just teenagers so you have to expect that". Are ALL two year olds and teenagers like that or are there ones that aren't? What are the statistics of the ones that fall into that category? Just saying? I have one child that probably did fit a little into that category and one that didn't. Was it where they were sleeping? In my case and knowing what I now know, I would say the answer is yes. One bedroom had one wall affected by GS and the other room had everything going on in it.

I have a client who as a young adolescent would often wake up during the night needing to go to the bathroom and was always angry! He wanted to punch walls and was basically angry at the world and whoever came his way. Was that because of where he slept? Could the location of his bed really cause such dramatic mood changes? Or was he going to be like that anyway? What if it was his location for most of his life? Where he had chosen (or was chosen for him) to sleep, with GS irritating him to the point of wanting to smash something.

After I dowsed his room it did turn out that he indeed had GS crossing his head while in bed.

It can have that effect on people, and maybe animals as well, especially animals in cages!

By moving his sleeping location only slightly he started sleeping through the night without waking. It calmed him, and his personality certainly settled down. He had more energy but in a good way, and wanted to get up and do healthy things with his life. Now years later those signs of regular aggression are nowhere to be seen.

Surely that is enough to make you want to know if there is any GS affecting anyone in your family who suffers with aggression or sudden irritability, doesn't it?

What if you are on the receiving end?

AUTO-IMMUNE DISEASE:

In all the cases I have come across over the last 20 years, where an auto-immune disease was present in a person, GS was also badly affecting the body. The people had either been sleeping or working over it for a long period of time or they were on a 'knot'. This is where two lines cross which creates a very strong amount of vibrating energy.

GS doesn't cause any of these issues, but what it does is it lowers your immune system so your body is unable to fight off disease.

Geopathic influences may be among the most neglected contributing or causative agents for cancer or other disease, especially auto-immune disease.

BABY CRYING A LOT/WON'T SETTLE:

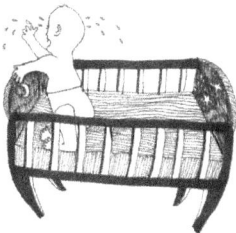

Well firstly mums and dads if this is your baby, give yourself a medal.

97

There is nothing worse than having a baby that won't settle, especially if it's your first. You poor things. There is nothing that anyone can say that helps. Of course when it's your first, you feel like you are the first person that has EVER been through anything like this and I know because I've been there. But believe me you are not alone.

First check:

- ✓ Are they hungry?
- ✓ Do they need their nappy changed?
- ✓ Do they have pain, like a bubble (wind) in their tummy or similar.

Once you have done all the obvious checks look at where you are putting them?

- ✓ Are you putting them in the cot or bassinet where they never really settle?

Or is this the pram in the lounge or wherever you happen to be.

Perhaps there is an invisible 'Energy' that is making this a 'BBP' (Bad Bed Position).

Take notice when they go down if they seem to quickly wriggle or start crying.

Or do they drop off to sleep but then don't stay asleep very long and wake irritated or crying?

You must make it a priority to know that the 'space' where you are about to put your angel or if you have twins or more 'angels', must be in a GS clear space. (We have lessons on how to do this later)

TWINS NOT SLEEPING FOR 5 YEARS:

Funnily I have a couple of stories about twins. One Mum had twins that NEVER slept through the night. She seriously needed a medal. It took 5 years before they finally started to sleep through the night. She and her partner would spend every night trying to amuse the twins as they would never settle. They would go for drives late at night or push them in their prams and then they would finally fall asleep. But when they came home and put them in their respective beds they would be irritated and wake up again. She used to say they needed stimulation so would spend all night reading to them or trying to pacify them, but nothing worked. She was exhausted.

At no point did they ever associate it with the location of their beds.

They finally started school and she had always suspected they needed more and that their brains just needed extra stimulation. When they started school they finally started sleeping though the night.

Guess what else happened?

They moved house, as they out grew their first small house.

Could their location have been causing all those sleepless nights?

TWINS: ONE SLEEPS, ONE DOESN'T

Rachel bought her two baby boys home and quickly noticed one baby boy slept and the other didn't.

It didn't take long before she also noticed one developed health issues, the other didn't. This included skin issues, allergies and food intolerances. By the way, the one that slept through the night is not the one that had the health issues.

Could the location of their beds really have caused such a dramatic difference in these two babies?

After dowsing their house it was identified where the boy that had the allergies, had also slept in several places in the small bedroom and all were affected by the same two lines of Geopathic noxious energy. How could it be the location of his cot as they had moved his bed 4 times?

The other twin that had no health issues had always slept in the same 'GS clear' position.

Rachel had tried moving the affected boy's cot and decided this was a better option than just swapping their beds. What if she ended up with two babies not sleeping. As a new Mum that option seemed terrifying.

So be careful just moving the bed around to see if you can find a clear space as you could 'jump out of the frying pan and into the fire'! Have a professional dowser come and check your

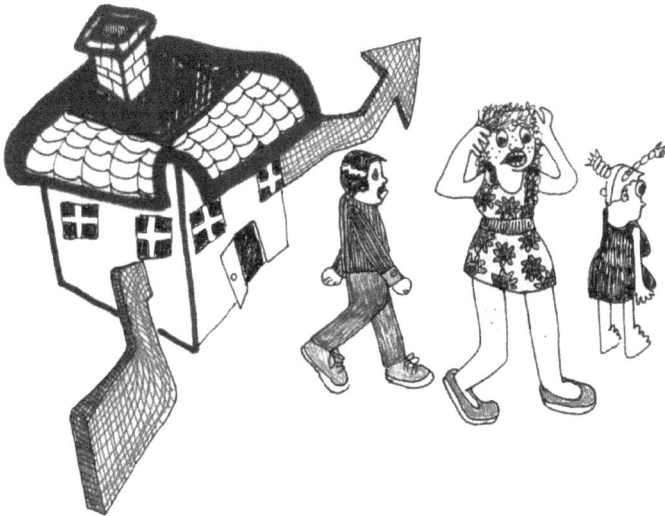

house before you bring your baby home from hospital. Or even more importantly when you are pregnant. Even better, before you decide to get pregnant.

Don't forget you can learn the 'gift' of dowsing later in the book.

BABY CRYING, DRIVING PARENTS CRAZY

Another story is of a little baby who had recently moved into a new house with his Mum and Dad. From the very first night this little boy did not settle and each night he would wriggle around in his bed and was completely disrupted. He would cry and cry and eventually his Mum would have to get him out of his bassinet and bring him into their bed with them. The Mum was at the end of her tether and being her first child, she had nothing to compare with so wondered if it was the smells of the new house or something else. Nothing made sense.

It didn't take long before the little boy got very sick and full of the flu as his immune system was compromised and he was very congested.

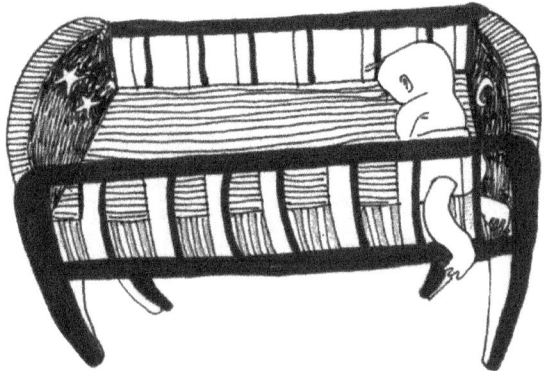

I had dropped some flyers in the area and she thought she had nothing to lose so would give it a try. As always I didn't know anything before I went in and just dowsed through as normal.

I found a GS line running directly up the entire length of his bed. The baby would instinctively need to get away from this energy and the direction it was flowing would push him around the bassinet. This of course was making him uncomfortable and as there was nowhere to escape to so he cried as you do when you're uncomfortable.

When Mum lifted him out of the bassinet, she unknowingly moved him off the Geopathic Stress, so it felt comfortable again and he could go straight back to sleep.

We moved the bassinet and within a few days, his immune system was strong again, his flu symptoms had all subsided and he was sleeping through the night, and now life goes on as it should with a sleeping baby.

Would every other Mum out there that has experienced 'sleepless nights' want this magic to happen to them?

I think so!

Stay tuned and we can help with that. We will help 'tune in' to your intuition or get professional dowser to help you.

BED WETTING:

The National Sleep Foundation Children's Hospital in Boston USA, have done research into bedwetting and have found that between 12-20% of 5 year olds wet the bed. There are also

10% of 7year olds and 5% of 10 year olds, or older, that also still wet the bed.

That is 5 to 7 million children in the United States alone still wet the bed on a regular basis. This accounts for 10% of the whole population of children in the US.

What if they are like my daughter (who I have to thank again for helping me understand this phenomenon called Geopathic Stress) who wet the bed until around 12years of age. It was not her fault Yet I'm sure I used to blame her. I didn't know any better. I just figured she could or should have stopped by now. Why was she doing it and not her brother? We tried to use alarms, 'time-out', monitors, charts, staying up late and everything else the experts at the time recommended.

However NO ONE, not doctors, specialists, parents, family or friends knew the answer. They also didn't know about these noxious energies.

Not one single person suggested all I needed to do was move the bed!

All I needed to do was identify where the Geopathic Stress was in her room and move her bed away from it. We had moved her bed over the years, but once we finally identified where these lines were, we were actually making it worse in the previous locations.

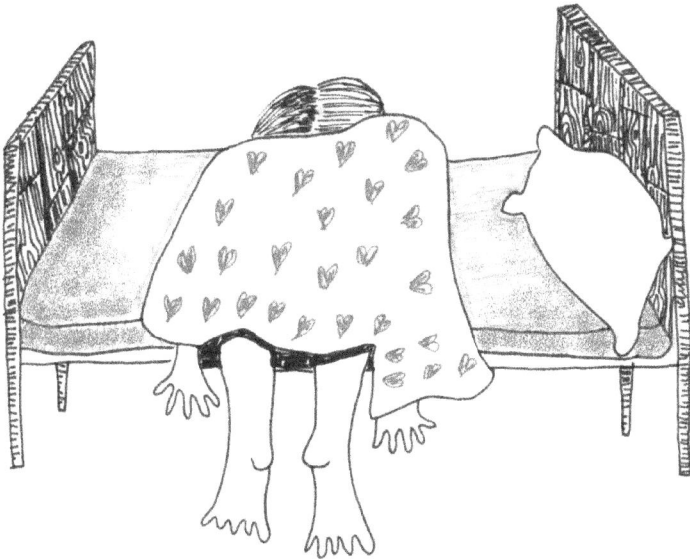

The poor little thing, no wonder she was a 'messy' sleeper always moving around a lot in her bed and often even waking on the floor. She never wanted to go to bed, yet her brother was fine with that.

"Why can't you be like your brother"? I'm sure I used to say. She couldn't be like him, because his bed was in a good, clear safe 'GS' free zone so he LIKED going to bed as it felt clear, nice and comfortable.

She on the other hand, felt tormented and irritated. So when she got into bed, she couldn't settle. Once she finally fell into an exhausted sleep she either couldn't wake up, or the vibration caused by the movement of this underground energy that was affecting her room was irritating her to the point of bed-wetting.

There was no conscious part of her body that knew this was going on, but it did affect her.

Again my darling, I am sorry for not knowing. Now is the time to make sure no other parents and especially a child has to go through what we went through.

BLOOD NOSE:

I have had several clients whose blood noses were definitely linked with where they were sleeping. One teenage boy, would wake up on a regular basis with a blood nose. His doctors couldn't explain why this was happening. After dowsing the house I identified a 'knot' where two lines cross directly on his pillow. I asked his Mum if he had trouble sleeping? She confirmed he not only had terrible trouble sleeping and nightmares, but also woke on a regular basis in the mornings with a blood nose.

Once I moved his bed, he not only slept through the night, but the nightmares stopped, and so did the nose bleeds.

CANCER:

Studies by Geomancers and Dowsers have shown over the years startling discoveries about the link between Cancer and Geopathic Stress.

Now these studies have been written off by the 'Cancer' Societies around the world as many Geomancers have tried to reach out to them with these discoveries.

However there is still a lot of evidence that shows if you have cancer or have it in your family you might like to take note of this info.

In 1929 a man called Gustav Von Pohl mapped out all the Geopathic Stress in a town called Vilsbiburg in Germany. There had been a lot of people die of cancer in this town and was asked to investigate. With a police guard he 'dowsed' through the village with no prior knowledge of where the people had died and marked on the map of the village the exact houses that the people had died of cancer. All 53 cases.

He could also identify what sort of cancer they had by where the Geopathic Stress ran through the bed location.

He later commented that 'Cancer was a disease of location'!

There are many others over the years that also have found significant links between Geopathic Stress and Cancer.

Geopathic influences may be among the most neglected contributing or causative agents for cancer and other disease. An official confirmation and endorsement was published in 1985 by Dr. Veronika Carstens MD (wife of the former German Federal President Karl Carstens): Dr. Carstens authored a study stating that there were 700 documented cases worldwide where terminal cancer patients had regained their health without any conventional treatment after their sleeping area had been moved from a geopathic stress zone. All of these cancer patients had been 'given up on' by their doctors. (Article from www.nlcare.org).

Geopathic Stress has been found to be the common factor in most serious and long-term illnesses and psychological conditions.

Scientists at *Dulwich Health Society, UK, studied over 25,000 people with ill health and concluded that the following groups are Geopathically Stressed (GS)

- ✓ 100% of people who get Secondary Cancer.
- ✓ 95% of people who get Cancer were sleeping & or working in a GS place before or at the time cancer was diagnosed.
- ✓ 95% of children who are Hyperactive, Learning Difficulties or are difficult to control.
- ✓ 95% of people who get AIDS.

- ✓ 80% of parents/caregivers who Abuse Children.
- ✓ 80% of Divorces are by one or both partners being Geopathically Stressed.
- ✓ 80% of couples whom Cannot Have Babies, one or both are on GS.
- ✓ 80% of women who have a miscarriage.
- ✓ 80% of babies who died of Cot Death
- ✓ 70% of M.E. (Post Viral Fatigue) sufferers.
- ✓ 70% of people who are Allergic to Food or Drink.

I find these statistics amazing and completely accurate. In the hundreds and hundreds of homes I have dowsed over the last 20 years, the same statistics have applied. This is in no way subliminal as I never know anything before I go in yet I get the same results.

CASE STUDY I: VICTORIA:

I went to Victoria's house and knew before I arrived that there was an issue with cancer, but that was all I knew. (Normally I don't like to know anything before I go to a house).

I started in the lounge and detected a GS line running through the room,

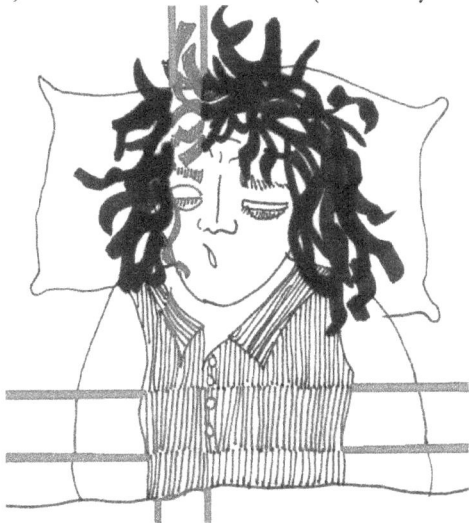

and disappeared into the wall (heading towards the bedrooms).

I walked down the hallway and picked up two other lines crossing this one. One crossed about the wall and didn't affect any furniture, but the next one crossed nearly at the end of the hallway. When I went into the master bedroom, the two lines crossed and formed a 'knot' on the middle upper right of the bed.

I asked Vicky who slept there, and she said she did. I told her that if anyone slept in this location, pointing to where the knot was forming on the bed, they would have major issues in the right breast side of the body.

She then informed me that she indeed had breast cancer in her right breast. It turned out she also didn't sleep well since she had moved into that house a year earlier.

The same line that crossed her upper body, continued into her daughters room across the hallway.

She also didn't sleep well and woke several times each night since she was born nearly 3 years ago.

We moved both the beds immediately, Vicky noticed her sleep improved straight away even after going through extensive treatments and having adverse effects from those treatments.

If you are able to have a good GS free sleep each night your body will start to do the healing needed while you are asleep. If

Geopathic Stress is zapping you every night, then your body gets no 'peace' and it will struggle to heal itself.

Several months later she called to inform me that her MRI had come up 'all clear', apart from slight scarring left over, which they were not concerned about. Here is what she said:

"I was diagnosed in July 2015 with breast cancer, through my alternative treatment I was having I was introduced to Nicky, who I am ever so grateful to have met. She came over and dowsed my home. I told her nothing and after showing me where the energy lines ran directly across the top of my chest and the other down the right side of my body (which is where the cancer was).

The one that ran through my chest also ran through my daughter's room and she had one that ran down the bottom of her bed. This was crazy because we had lived there a whole year and she had never slept through the night. She would wake 2-4 times a night.

I would have to get up at least 5-6 times before I could settle and sleep , then would always wake up feeling crap.

We had to move my daughter's room to the toy room and re arrange my room. It took a few days for my daughter to settle and now she sleeps through the night. I also have the best sleeps that I have had in a long time. Even though at the time I was having chemo and was sick, I still had peaceful sleeps.

Victoria, Auckland New Zealand.

Victoria was trying everything and did all she could to get rid of this cancer, but you can do all the right things, eat right with fresh and raw fruits and vegetables, exercise appropriately for your body, take the supplements and vitamins your body needs along with other treatments necessary, including drugs if required, but if you go and sleep in a GS zone or have one crossing your workspace, you are going 'one step forward and two steps backwards' each night.

If your body is compromised already with cancer, then the Geopathic Stress will speed up the process.

CASE STUDY II: CLAIRE

Another cancer case I had was for the daughter of a lady who had sadly passed away the year previous of a cancerous tumor in her head.

She wanted me to check the house to make sure that it was ok for her Dad who was still living in the home.

I went down the hallway, having never been in the house previously and found a line well before the entrance to the bedroom further down the hallway.

I then continued to walk and found no more lines that were crossing this room.

I walked past the room to see if I could find anything else and located a line that sharply turned back and crossed this empty room.

Entering the room, which was filled with a few boxes and no sign of any bed I found where the two lines 'knotted' or crossed.

On identifying this the lady was quite emotional as the parents had only two years earlier moved the bed to this location and the 'knot' crossed directly where her mother's head would have been when sleeping in the bed. She died of a brain tumor.

Coincidence? Possibly, but to identify exactly where her Mother had been sleeping for the last two years with no signs in the room of a bed or any other furniture to help, and for her to have a brain tumor exactly where this 'knot' was located is scary to say the least.

What if she had not moved her bed to that position? Could she still be alive?

Sadly we will never know but you need to know where these energies are in your home so you can avoid them.

CELIAC/COELIAC DISEASE/DIGESTION ISSUES:

Celiac disease -- also known as celiac sprue or Coeliac disease, or gluten-sensitive enteropathy -- is a digestive and autoimmune disorder that results in damage to the lining of the small intestine when foods with gluten are eaten. Gluten is a form of protein found in some grains. Every time I find my clients with these conditions, they have Geopathic Stress either where they sleep or where they are spending time stationary. If it is at your work, and you sit at a desk or spend time either standing or sitting and Geopathic Stress is crossing your body then your whole torso will be affected, especially your digestive system.

The first thing that happens when we eat is our digestive system kicks into processing the food. So if an irritation vibration caused by GS is present in your digestive system area, then it can't do what it is supposed to be doing which is to process the food and drink, you've sent down.

It is such a delicate system and a foreign irritation like GS will only cause problems.

Make sure before you change your whole life and your diet (not saying a gluten free diet is bad), make sure that is the issue first and it's not Geopathic Stress that is causing your gut issues.

CHILD LEUKEMIA:

This is similar obviously to 'Cancer' but of the blood and in children. As I have already mentioned before, children are even more sensitive to this energy than adults are.

So it would make sense that if geopathic stress affects us and has been found in studies that have been done on cases of cancer showing 95% of people studied that had cancer, were sleeping in a Geopathically stressed location. But scarily 100% of cases of people with secondary degree cancer were on a GS zone.

This is interesting:

Dr. A (a naturopathic physician) has this to say: "The cancer patient needs to relocate –FAST!

As early as the 1930's, world-famous German surgeon Professor Dr. Med. Ferdinand Sauerbruch told all his cancer patients NEVER return to their habitual sleeping place. For centuries it has been known that certain houses have a much higher incidence of cancer, arthritis, multiple sclerosis and many other degenerative diseases. Only in the 1970's was a satisfactory answer found; these diseases are due to geopathogenic zones, which usually are caused by a conversion of gravity field energy from radioactive radiation, electromagnetic phenomena in the neighborhood of subterranean streams or even high power lines or color TV's. Many times, a good dowser can locate these anomalies and appropriate measures can be taken to correct the situation.

As a first step, avoid the use of electric blankets, waterbeds, hair dryers and any electric influences that generate an electrical field of 60 hertz (cycles per second). Only if the patient is removed from these potentially damaging zones, does he/she have a maximum chance of permanent and speedy recovery in conjunction with diet, lifestyle and psychological modifications.

It may be a bit presumptuous to say that the above-mentioned geopathical zones CAUSE cancer, however, it is possible that they CONTRIBUTE to the causation of cancer" Reference from www.healingcancernaturally.com

CROHNS DISEASE:

Crohns Disease attacks the Digestive system, anywhere between the Mouth and the Anus. Generally the wrong types of food can irritate the gut and create the symptoms associated with Crohns. Stress is also a big contributor. My son developed Crohns Disease in his early 20's and there is no question in my mind that it was bought on by the location of his bed for the 18months prior to it being diagnosed. For the record I dowsed the property when we bought it and I even had another 'dowser' come and verify what I had found. However as teenagers do he moved his room around a little and moved his bed only half a metre to one side, which put him directly in the line of Geopathic Stress (underground water). For the next 12 to18 months it seriously irritated him. He would moan that his bed was uncomfortable and he needed a new bed. He would always ask me to massage his back as it was so sore. He would always get very aggressive and angry. I thought it was attributed to his age and blamed the stress of University.

Now if it was anyone else I would have identified it immediately. You know the old story of the 'Plumber' having a leaking tap at home, or the 'Builder' with the unfinished building work on his own house.

I was too close to see.

After the surgeon sadly told my son "He has a DISEASE called Crohns and would have it for the rest of his life" - his exact words. (Some Doctor's really do need a better bedside manner).

I immediately thought Geopathic Stress and Crohns, could there be a link? I had never heard of Crohns and didn't even know how to spell it at the time. I went to dowse his room and he asked if he could do it himself as he can dowse. He straightaway identified the line running from head to feet along his bed. It was running directly through his gut.

We moved the bed immediately and within a week or so the same bed that was causing him pain before wasn't hurting his back anymore, and he was at least sleeping better.

Because the time he had spent there had caused serious damage to his digestive system, drugs were needed to stabilize the situation.

7 years on he is doing amazing. He is very aware if he is not sleeping and will move his bed or have me dowse it when he changes locations.

How many other people are out there blaming the food they are eating or stress on the issues like Crohns, Celiac, or IBS, instead of identifying if GS is the cause and moving the bed.

CHRONIC FATIGUE:

85% of Chronic Illnesses are linked with Geopathic Stress.

Wow what a statement, but what if it is true?

I have found that in all the cases I have dowsed over the last 20 years, that if a chronic illness was present so was Geopathic Stress.

When I dowse, I never know what issues people have or where they sleep. I ask them not to tell me. However I will identify where in the body there is a likelihood of something being wrong by where the Geopathic Stress is crossing the bed or wherever else they spend time stationary.

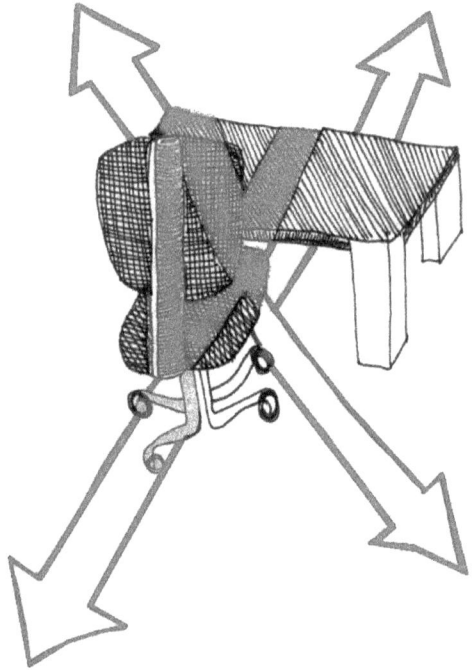

I went to dowse the home of a friend of mine who was

diagnosed with Chronic Fatigue many years ago. Before I went there I 'did' in this instance know he had been diagnosed with this and when I dowsed his room, expecting to find GS in his bed even though I wasn't aware what side he slept on, the whole bed was relatively ok. A line was close to one side, but I wasn't worried about it.

I then dowsed his office, which is where he spent up to 8 hours a day at his desk. Directly on his chair was a very strong 'knot'. (Where two lines cross)

The rest of the family informed me that whenever they sat at the desk, they would feel uncomfortable or have the urge to go to the toilet often.

The desk was moved immediately.

Now 12 years on, and a healthy lifestyle 'no geopathic stress', he is fitter and healthier than ever.

DIARRHEA/CONSTIPATION:

If you are having trouble with diarrhea or constipation check where you are sleeping or 'sitting' during the day? Again we are talking about part of the whole digestive system.

If you are 'sitting' in the wrong place your whole body could be affected. This will attack that part of your body (your torso sitting on the chair or standing) and lower the ability for your body to do its job. I have had cases of people affected by GS where they sat at work and it started with Diarrhea and/or constipation and went on to develop into Bowel Cancer. Also make sure you are drinking lots of water.

Move where you are sitting, before it moves you…

DEPRESSION:

The normal ups and downs of life mean that everyone feels sad or has 'the blues' from time to time. But if emptiness and despair have taken hold of your life and won't go away you may have depression.

Depression makes it tough to function and enjoy life like you once did. Just getting through the day can be overwhelming. But no matter how hopeless you feel you can get better. Understanding the signs and symptoms is the first step to overcoming the problem. Sometimes for people the signs are not that clear especially when you have depression. It is easy to blame it on everything else that is going on around you. Sometimes you feel that no one 'gets you' and they just don't understand what is happening to you.

SOPHIE'S STORY: Here is a story about one of my customers Sophie (not her real name) who first showed me how Geopathic Stress and Depression are so completely connected. I also want to say thank you to her as your example has helped me help so many others over the years!

Sophie was around 15years old but small in stature, and had been living in the family house for 10 years. She had always been in the same bedroom, either she chose it or was given when they arrived. This room had some serious Geopathic Stress affecting the bedroom and creating a knot directly on her bed. This was generating GS up to 200 times more than what is healthy for her body. It was so bad there was nowhere else to safely put her bed to be clear of it as it, was such a small bedroom. She had not been to school for 18 months and was being home schooled as she was too sick to attend.

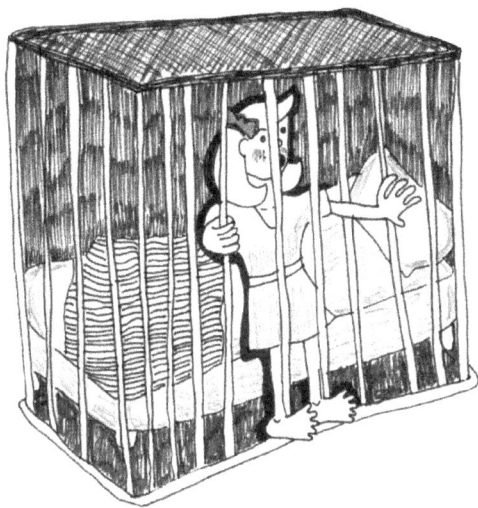

For me the 'negative energy' in her room was so strong that it was like she was living in 'a cage' around her bed, with a big 'knot' right in the middle, she agreed and said had been telling all her councilors but no one believed her.

Then she said she just couldn't reach her hand out to get the key!

Now sadly, her little body had almost got used to this 'noxious earth energy'! It is a bit like a smoker, you know it's not good for you but you just can't keep away from it.

It had become comfortable and familiar even though it was seriously irritating her.

The option I could see was to move her out of this room to a larger room with her sister.

She had two little budgies that were in the room with her (in the only clear space in the room), that were also being affected by the 'heavy' feeling in this room.

We put them outside on the balcony, and they seemed to flourish.

Sophie was moved into another room in the house and a week later I rang to see how things were going and was told that she had felt well enough to go to school that day.

How many other children and adults are on 'drugs' to help them cope with depression, that simply need to check the bedroom where they spend each night isn't making them feel even more depressed.

There is the probability it develops into a vicious circle as you feel so bad you can't move away from it, and because you feel bad you don't have the energy to do anything about it.

*Depression is a serious condition and I am in no way saying this is the answer to all the cases, but it sure is a good place to start. If you start with the places you spend the most time it will give you a reasonable idea. Of course with depression many people feel the need to stay on the couch or in their bed as they have no will power to move. This could be yet another 'location based' illness, or at least aggravated by the location.

You should notice quickly if you start sleeping better then you might start feeling better, or at least have the will to try.

DIZZINESS/NAUSEA:

You tend to notice this quite quickly if you cross a GS zone. It is generally in one of the first stages of the 'Six stages of Geopathic Stress'.

You might have this when you walk through a large 'knot' as this will give you a dizzy feeling and certainly can make you feel nauseous. I have had it when I have gone to the movies or sat down at a restaurant for dinner and will feel it very quickly, and recognize that I am sitting in a GS Zone. Easy fix - MOVE. Don't stay there, as it won't get better only worse.

The thing is in the past you probably would have 'stayed' there and then it has worsened, so then you took anti-nausea pills, or you felt so bad that you had to go and lie down. Of course as long as you have a nice clear sleeping place you will start to feel better quite quickly. But what if this is where you sit at work?

What if this is your favourite place to sit at University, or School? Or you are the boss, or Prime Minister what happens then?

Do you just right it off to 'that's how you often feel', and take drugs to make you feel better.

Do you feel so bad that you have to leave your job? (This did happen to one of my clients).

If it is where you sit while you are studying then it could affect your concentration and it will have a snowball affect on your general learning and health. At least make sure it is not something as simple as 'sitting in the wrong place'!

ECZEMA/PSORIASIS:

I have been plagued with Psoriasis since I was a child. I remember having to sit while my mother applied this horrible 'stinky' tar ointment all over my body. At various stages in my life it reappeared "Oh well it's in my family, so this is my lot"!

I always thought it was funny how it was only my sister, mother and myself that had it, not my Brother or Father. We moved around a lot as we were growing up, and when I look back, I had it at some houses and not at others.

I NEVER associated it with Geopathic Stress or my location until about 20 years ago, when I thought back to where I was sleeping 2 years before being diagnosed with Chronic Arthritis. I also had 'Raindrop Psoriasis' all over my body.

For those of you that don't know what that is it was hard to put a dot between them. I was covered and they looked like polka-dots.

I didn't link the two but now 20 years on and always aware of where the GS is in my home, I don't have regular bouts of psoriasis. I have had it about 5 times in the last 20 years, in the winter when not out in the sun as you are in summer. But only one or two small dots appear. Nothing even close to what I used to get.

I put some coconut oil or similar on them and they disappear. To be fair the sun is the best thing for them in my opinion.

Considering I have had it in some form for the last 50 plus years I feel qualified to comment. Thankfully I am currently clear of it.

ENDOMETRIOSIS/PMS:

I was diagnosed with chronic endometriosis about 15 years ago and had to have two operations to remove it. This was over period of 5 years. It was removed and then it returned. I never considered the link between where I was sleeping at the time

(Geopathic Stress) and this issue. It was early in my GS studies and I didn't consider it.

To be fair I was in so much pain I'm pretty sure my head wasn't thinking straight. A few years back I was remembering that situation and the other symptoms I was having at the time like constant cramps and aches and pains, including lower back pain and there is no question in my mind, that there is a connection between the two. We moved house and I never had any of those issues again.

GRINDING TEETH:

At the times in my life when things like Psoriasis and nightmares were affecting me, I was also grinding my teeth. My daughter also did this when she was wetting her bed. The children of several of my clients particularly those who were having sleep issues were also grinding their teeth at night. Is there a link? Worth checking don't you think. Much cheaper than a large dentist bill.

HEADACHES/MIGRAINES:

These often happen in the first stages as previously mentioned in the Six Stages of Geopathic Stress in Chapter One, and GS will irritate you quite

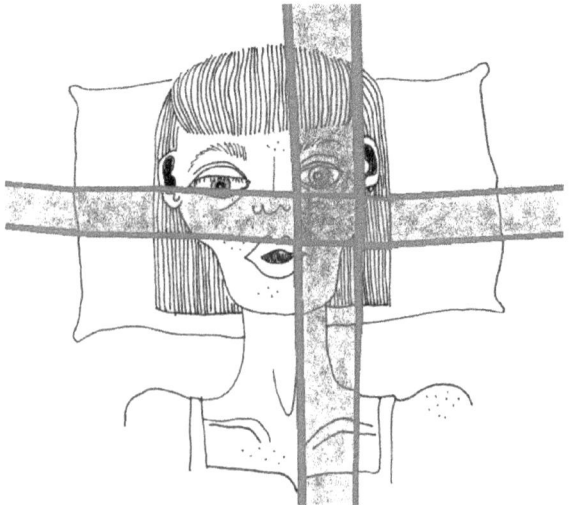

quickly. If you load on top of the situation EMF's (Electromagnetic Fields or Radiation), you will really be feeling it.

I recently did a remote dowsing at a clients house and identified a 'knot' crossing right on her side of the bed and pillow.

I asked her if she had trouble sleeping and woke with headaches. "All the time"! she said, and also had regular Migraines.

Mmmmmmm… Are you getting the picture? Don't forget one of the most common reasons for headaches is lack of water, so make sure you are very hydrated as well.

IBS/IRRITABLE BOWEL SYNDROME:

This is closely linked with Crohns/Celiac and digestive disorders which we have already covered, but because of our daily intake of food which goes directly into our digestive system, if your 'system' is being aggravated nightly by Geopathic Stress, it has no chance to cope with everything we put into it. So what's it going to do…chuck it out of your system, the quickest way possible?

LEARNING DIFFICULITIES/ADHD:

95% of cases relating to Children with ADHD and learning difficulties featured in several studies from the United

Kingdom and Germany are linked with GS.

A study done by Käthe Bachler* back in the early 70's, after researching more than 11,000 people in over 3,000 apartments, houses and work places in 14 countries, discovered the huge link between Geopathic Stress and children's learning problems.

She was a dowser and a teacher and noticed year after year the significance of the location in the classroom and the relativity to disruptive people.

Last year it was 'Little Johnny' (sorry to all the good Johnnies out there), and the next year it was 'Little Ted who was the class terror'. The common link was they were sitting in the same 'location' in the classroom so it made her wonder. Was the location significant?

 (*Earth Radiation by Käthe Bachler published by The Holistic Intuition Society).

LACK OF ENERGY:

If you wake up feeling tired after a full nights 'supposed' sleep, there is a good chance there could be a link between where you are sleeping, GS and this lack of energy.

Imagine your body gets into bed at night and is exhausted from your day's activities.

Then straight away it starts to feel the effects of GS. This can vary depending on how strong it is.

If you are on a knot (where two lines cross), it could be as high as 250hertz. This is over 200 times more than what is healthy for us for long periods of time. We want it to be around the 7.83hertz, which is the Schumann Resonance.

There is a narrow window between around 10pm and 2am when the Melatonin in your body are doing their best work.

Melatonin is produced in the pineal gland.

Melatonin is one of the most essential hormones in the body.

Previously it has been known as the 'darkness hormone', as the levels rise only ever at night.

One of its purposes is to signal the body that its night time, and also perform its specialised functions during this time, which is synergistic with sleep.

Melatonin is also a powerful anti-oxidant and improves our immune function which is why it often has an 'anti-cancer' title.

It's main purpose is to regulate the 'circadian rhythm'. This daily rhythmic activity cycle is based on a 24-hour interval, which is exhibited by many organisms including humans.

It is so important because this clock tells our bodies the best time to do things like sleep, eat and exercise.

Of course at night when it is dark and the sun is on the other side of the Earth i.e. your location, this is when your body can do its best healing.

Over a 24 hour period our body has certain 'jobs' it does at certain times.

The Circadian rhythms, according to 'Google' are: Physical, mental and behavioral changes that follow a roughly 24-hour cycle, responding primarily to light and darkness in an organism's environment.

They are found in most living things including animals, plants and many tiny microbes.

The study of **circadian rhythms** is called '**chronobiology'.**

A rough look at this in a 24 hour period looks a little like this:

- Midnight –

- 2am   Deepest Sleep

- 4.30am   Lowest body temperature

- 6.45am   Sharpest Rise in Blood Pressure

- 7.30am   Melatonin secretion stops

- 8.30am   Bowel movement likely

- 9am   Highest testosterone secretion

- 10am   High alertness

- Midday

- 2.30pm   Best co-ordination

- 3.30pm   Fastest reaction time (time to step up to the mark)

- 5pm   Greatest cardiovascular efficiency and muscle strength

- 6pm   Highest blood pressure

- 7pm   Highest body temperature

- 9pm   Melatonin secretion starts (that's why its good to go to bed early)

- 10.30pm   Bowel movements suppressed.

If at any of these crucial times you are being zapped by GS while you 'think' you are sleeping, instead of healing and rejuvenating like they are supposed to all the cells in your body will be struggling.

Hence when you wake in the morning you WILL literally be exhausted because the cells didn't get the rest they needed to help you heal, grow and strengthen for your next day.

Don't blame the pillow or the bed until you have at least checked that GS is not present.

Of course I understand and accept there are many other things that can cause lack of sleep such as STRESS. Just don't let it be Geopathic STRESS.

HIGH & LOW BLOOD PRESSURE:

This is a common illness in the Twenty First Century. The change in blood sugars and blood pressure can kick in as early as the third stage of Geopathic Stress. If your body is being irritated by the vibration of GS, especially near the area of your heart then it will go into 'defense mode' to protect your body by either lowering or raising your blood pressure to cope.

A person will react depending on the intensity of their Geopathic Stress situation.

It will depend on what stage they are at considering how long they have been affected. By the time it is close to causing blood pressure issues you will have no doubt already had trouble with sleeping problems, lack of concentration, exhaustion, back pain, allergies and possibly migraines.

With this constant irritation from GS, illness will increase including high blood pressure, asthma, diabetes and chronic skin diseases. If left undetected the body's immune system will be seriously compromised and severe diseases such as cancer can manifest.

MENOPAUSE/PMS:

What if the monthly periods women have are exacerbated by where you are sleeping? I have an interesting scenario where my mother had extremely bad monthly periods and also menopause issues including chronic hot sweats. Yet I have breezed through the whole experience, without noticing anything.

Is there a chance that where she slept either at the point of puberty or any other time in her life could have aggravated the situation? We moved around a lot and maybe some places were worse than others?

My daughter also experienced far more severe issues than I did and I 'know' she was being affected where she was sleeping during puberty.

Just a thought!

I also know for sure that some people experience the symptoms of Geopathic Stress as 'hot or cold' feelings so if you are going through Menopause and every night you go to bed and experience really bad 'hot flushes' make sure it isn't GS that is heating you up.

MISCARRIAGE/COT DEATH:

80% of cases of Miscarriages and cot deaths have been linked with the presence of GS. Several of my client cases have had trouble getting pregnant or have sadly lost a baby, and when I dowsed the location I identified that the GS is directly where they were sleeping or placed the cot. The frequency, well over the 7.83hertz of the Schumann resonance, could be as high as 100-226htz. This is too high for an embryo or a baby. NASA acknowledges this frequency by putting 'Schumann Resonators' in its capsules, when they send astronauts to space.

It is much easier for us. All we need to do is 'check where it is in your home' and don't put a bed or a cot there.

If you are being affected when you are pregnant what else could it do to the baby?

I don't know, it's just a thought.

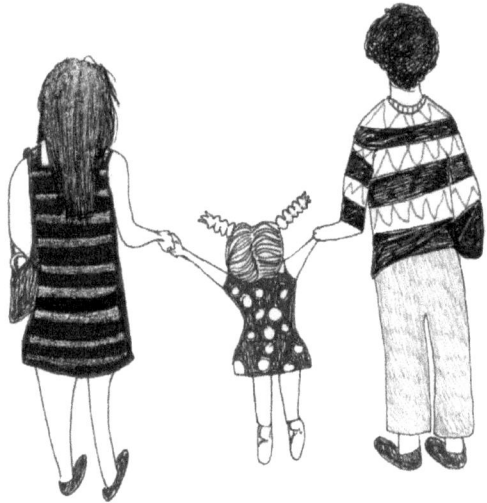

Here's an interesting thought. How many times have you heard of people who can't have children and decide to adopt. Then once they have a adopted they get pregnant on their own. How many of these people MOVED either their bed, bedroom or moved house?

Just saying!

PREGNANCY ISSUES/TROUBLE FALLING PREGNANT:

With statistics of previous studies as high as 80% of cases of miscarriages being linked to GS, then of course the same applies to having trouble even falling pregnant. You imagine the tiny embryo having to deal with the frequencies of Geopathic Stress being as high as 200 times what is necessary for us, then it's understandable that this will cause a problem.

Over the years I have had numerous cases of people trying to get pregnant without success then moving the bedroom around and falling pregnant very quickly. I am excited to be catching up with a newborn baby this week where that is exactly the case. So you see how important it is to know where these energies are for you as parent trying to get pregnant and for the baby after it is born.

SLEEP DISORDERS:

During wartime people have used Sleep Deprivation as a form

of torture. Sadly we are doing this to ourselves every night if you choose to sleep in a GS zapped zone. Either get your home tested or learn from this book, how to test it for yourself.

Make sure you are not torturing yourself nightly!

STOMACH ULCERS:

These are also linked with 'digestive' issues. When we are stressed many people will take it straight to their gut. We eat daily so therefore it is the likely place for disturbance to happen, especially if your gut is already getting a zap from GS somewhere in your day. Could be at night in your bed or could be on the couch. Is it at your desk at work? What if you stand up all day and still have an issue?

Are you frequently standing in the same place? I remember hearing of a case many years ago in Australia where they closed down a Post Office because a significant number of the female staff developed 'breast cancer'. They were standing in the 'tellers' positions as long as many people sit at their desk.

After testing they found a line of GS running lengthwise where all the ladies were standing for hours on end, day after day. They called it 'sick building syndrome'.

I call it GEOPATHIC STRESS.

If the architect had someone 'dowse' for GS before deciding where to put the counters or where people were going to stand all day, it could have saved their lives and the subsequent closing of the building as it was condemned as unsafe.

UNEASY FEELINGS/HOT AND COLD SENSATIONS:

Have you ever walked into a room and had an uneasy feeling or even felt a sudden hot or cold feeling? In my experience I notice where the GS 'knots' are and there is often an uneasy feeling associated with it. This may spook a few people, and it can also be where 'spirits' are present. The knot can act as a pot-hole, and spirits, ghosts, entities, or whatever you want to call them can enter. They may or may not be there to see you and may just be passing through, but that is a whole different book. Check out 'Spirit Release' A Practical Handbook, by Sue Allen.

WEIGHT-GAIN OR LOSS:

Think about it. If it's hard to get out of bed it's going to make it hard to get moving. What if GS is zapping your favourite couch or chair? It doesn't really make you want to leap out of bed and get moving does it? Feeling lethargic is one of the definite signs of GS. As stated previously it drains you. No way do you want to get out and get moving.

Have you moved into a house and then put on weight?

Do you sleep well? Just saying, it could be linked.

137

Here are some illnesses and diseases that have been linked with Geopathic Stress.

- Headaches

- Anxiety

- Dizziness

- Nightmares

- Child Leukemia

- Loss of Sex Drive

- Lack of Appetite

- Arthritis & Rheumatic Disorders

- Inability to concentrate

- Heart disease – of all types

- Hypersensitivity to light

- Leukemia and Lymphomas

- Irritability

- Feeling cold

- Tingling in arms and legs

- Grinding teeth

- Suicide

- Multiple sclerosis

- Motor neuron disease

- Premature birth

- Unhealthy new-born babies – including:

- Down's syndrome

- Failure to thrive

- Hyperactivity

- Difficult to control

- Panic Attacks

- Anorexia

- Loss of Appetite

- Exhaustion after very little physical or mental exertion

- Parkinson's disease

- Lack of patience
- Asthma
- Insomnia
- Addictions
- Restless sleep
- Marriage disharmony/breakups
- Sleep walking
- ADHD (Attention deficit disorder)
- Nightmares
- Allergies to drink, foods, or environmental triggers
- Chronic fatigue syndrome
- High blood pressure
- Stomach ulcers
- Aids
- Meningitis
- E. Coli food poisoning
- Loss of balance

- Short term memory loss

- Schizophrenia

- Obsessions

- Not wanting to go to bed

- Feeling better when away from home

- Emotional over-sensitivity

- Infertility (storks will not visit, let alone nest on a Geopathically stressed zone)

Even though this seems to be a huge list, these illnesses and diseases have been linked with Geopathic Stress in the United Kingdom, USA, Europe, Asia Pacific so it is in your best interest if you suffer any of these or know someone who is suffering from any of the above, then make sure you at least eliminate Geopathic Stress as possible cause.

Don't let all the other good work you are doing be held back by your location!

For example where you sleep, sit or stand as some people stand at a counter for just as long as many sit at a desk.

EVERYTHING FROM HEADACHES TO CANCER

This is Kimberley's story and it covers everything including headaches, blood noses, lack of energy, chronic fatigue, weight gain, insomnia, being unmotivated, nausea, ringing in the ears as well as prostrate and bone cancer. Not counting all the issues with their electrical appliances and this is just in two houses.

How many other people are out there are in exactly the same situation and just think they have 'bad luck'!

Kimberley tells it best:

'In 2014 my family and I relocated to rural Silverdale, north of Auckland, NZ. We chose the home and location because we felt it would be the best place to reside away from the congestions of EMF's. I felt at the time it was a healthy environment and would be a good place to live. Prior to moving, my son and I were very active and went to the gym 5-6 days per week. My Father of 86 also lived with us and used to walk to the beach and rode his bike to town daily. At the time, the only medication he took was for his blood pressure.

Soon after moving I began to slowly lose energy. I became moody and felt stressed. I also woke regularly with headaches. Toilet runs at night were also becoming more frequent. I was also experiencing weight gain even though my diet was the same and in fact I was eating less and better than ever.

My partner Murray was having big problems with chronic fatigue, nausea and extreme ringing in the ears. My father also had a very good diet, but even with the best of food and high quality supplements began to decline in both his health and energy rapidly. My 16year old son was waking up with headaches and soon began to suffer insomnia and regular nose bleeds. All of our conditions continued and worsened through the year. My son left to attend school overseas three months after moving in and shortly after arriving at school said his headaches and insomnia had improved. My father who remained with us slowly deteriorated and became so ill that he was unable to leave the house for days at a time. He spent most of his time in his bedroom sleeping. Murray (my partner) was unable to overcome the chronic fatigue and he too fell victim to the sleepless nights and excessive bed rest.

In February 2015 we acquired a holiday home in the township of Coromandel. After three visits to our new holiday home, both my partner and I woke up daily with extreme body pain and headaches. It was so intense that I was unable to function without at least 2-3 cups of very strong coffee. Strangely we were also experiencing ongoing issues with appliances in the kitchen and had replaced both our brand new washing machine and dishwasher. The refrigerator even though new, was having multiple issues.

I came across some information a few years back on Geopathic Stress. but dismissed it believing GS did not affect me, even though I had many of the symptoms on and off that were discussed in the article. After moving to our home in Silverdale and regular visits to our holiday home in the Coromandel there was no denying my gut feeling that there was something affecting us that was environmentally related. To my good fortune a dear friend of mine who knew what was happening referred me to Nicky.

The very next day I contacted her for a visit to our Coromandel home. Nicky requested that I not reveal any information to her prior to her coming to our property.

Her findings there were astonishing!

She first dowsed the main living area then the master bedroom where Murray and I had been sleeping. In that room she found 2 GS lines crossing on our bed, in the kitchen she found another 2 major GS lines. One right down the side where all our appliances are located and the other one ran through our pantry where we have been having problems with ants and rodents. Even though the pantry is not used for food storage we keep cleaning products and dishware in there.

I relocated the master bed to the back room where it is clear of GS and then moved the other beds to the front room away from the GS lines. Both Murray and I are pleased to report that for the first time, we slept very well and woke up free of body aches and headaches. I later remembered that the previous owner had passed away after getting sick in the house and he would have slept in the master bedroom, where we couldn't sleep.

A few weeks later I asked Nicky to come out to our home in Silverdale, again she asked not to be told anything. Her findings again were astonishing!

She found yet another crossing of geopathic stress lines meeting in the center of our master bed. In the room where my son use to sleep had a line directly across where his head rested. However the most tragic of all was the room where my father slept and spent most of his time. When Nicky tested his room she was not aware of any of the history or whose room it was, nor any of my father's health issues. The room was clear of all furniture, so she had no idea where the placement of his bed or other furnishings had been.

What she found was alarming! The room has three major GS lines crossing in a triangle directly located dead center where his bed once was. I then confessed to Nicky that about six months after moving to Silverdale my father was diagnosed with prostate and bone cancer. What is even more interesting is that only a few months before our move to that house my father had his annual PSA screening done at our local clinic in Whangamata. His levels were outstanding for a man of his age,

4ng.ml. However only after a few months in our new home he became ill and left New Zealand mid May 2015 to the US to seek treatment for prostrate and bone cancer. Also completely oblivious to it being the location that was causing my Fathers issues, Murray used that room for recuperation and having afternoon naps. One day I was looking for him and went into that room, and there he was in the middle of the day, sprawled out with his mouth open completely comatose, I almost mistook him for my Dad. It was very scary.

It has now been only six weeks since Nicky has evaluated our homes. I have placed the various energy bombs™ in all the recommended locations to absorb and soften GS. We have moved furniture according to her recommendations and I am happy to report that I have come though the GS detox period with an overall feeling of wellbeing and the return of my energy. I am no longer waking up with headaches and the frequent trips to the bathroom have lessened. Murray is also starting to come out of the haze and is feeling stronger both physically and emotionally. He has not needed an afternoon nap since. I am back to working out at the gym 4 days a week and home to resume to my normal works regime.

I definitely feel everyone should have their house checked and cleared of Geopathic Stress as it can have life changing results as it has done for us.

I highly recommend Nicky. Her work is remarkable. She explained everything she was doing in simple language and was great to ring us afterwards to see how everything was going and offer additional ongoing support. I love you Nicky! Murray and I are forever indebted to you!'

Kimberley Gabbard, Director, Prana NZ Ltd.

WHAT OTHERS HAVE TO SAY:

I have worked in the health industry for 20 years with clients that have had a huge range of issues, from pain, to diabetes, immune issues and cancer.

I first had Nicky in to find any lines of geopathic stress in my home. My youngest son now sleeps through the night and we all have more energy. Nicky then re-arranged my business premises. All our staff has noticed the difference, and clients keep commenting on the 'great energy'! I now send my family, friends and clients to Nicky and have seen every single person find benefit. From improved immune health and less sickness, to feeling happier and more energised.

This is a necessity in our modern society as a foundation of health. I cannot more highly recommend Nicky, her knowledge and techniques and am in awe of the 'Energy Bombs'™!

Susie Turner - BA Physical Geography, Owner Suna Pilates, Applied Kinesiology, Holistic Nutrition, TBM Practitioner, Auckland NZ.

I enlisted Nicky's help when I found I was having unusual trouble sleeping while visiting my Dads home. I sleep really well normally so this was really noticeable and constant enough that I didn't want to stay at his house. A friend referred me to Nicky, she came out to the property to diagnose the possible problem. As she will explain in her book there were very prominent lines running through the house in a manner in which were disrupting not only my sleep but my father's health. We were advised to move away from these lines especially where they ran through the bed. In my Dads case he was unaware as was I that one line ran through his bed at prostate, bowel and liver level, he had previously had bowel cancer and was experiencing urinary issues on occasions up 10x a night. His wife had recently died of liver cancer.

Nicky provides very clear down to earth explanations of what and why this is happening, I have since had my own home and business in Wellington cleared and balanced as well as my daughter's home in order for us all to maximize our health with as little interference as possible from this unseen but very influential force. As a Naturopath, herbalist and nurse I have experienced the full range of pros and cons that come with working in a field where not everything is visible - but the proof is in the pudding by treating the cause not just the symptoms we are all feeling alot better. I now sleep well with no strange unexplained disturbances. Thanks Nicky it has been a really interesting time.

<u>Amanda Haskell</u> -ND, EN, BHSc, Wellington, NZ

After a brain Aneurysm and associated stroke symptoms.

Nicky sourced the major areas where energy flow was affecting us in our home.
What a difference it has made to our general health and wellbeing. I have experienced a marked improvement in my health and no longer endure the pain and problems associated with colitis and, more importantly I have recovered from the brain surgery.

MB - Auckland, NZ

Since meeting Nicky & learning more about geopathic stress I have since noticed tingling in areas around the house and the behavior of our pets and plants. One plant I had inside struggling to grow is now doing amazingly well in its new spot.

Also our son had been getting up in the morning as if he had gone 10 rounds in the ring and was pumped up to go 10 more.
Nicky identified that there were 2 lines 'knotting' through his room and 1 outside. Note; this is not a big room.
We moved the bed into a clear space and put an energy bomb on the windowsill on the line of energy.
After 2 days he got out of bed calmer, more centered and more pleasant – let's be real he is a teenager. However he continued to get more and more calm and easy to be around. His inner bear seemed to be hybernating. His overall management of himself has improved hugely.

Carol Auckland – NZ

I'd moved six months prior and had been suffering with shoulder and hip pain on my right side not long after I'd moved. I thought it was as a result of excess weight training I was doing and was having weekly physio to fix it. But when Nicky mapped my place, she discovered my bed was on a Geopathic Stress line– right down my right side. Also I had not told her any of my symptoms before.

Within a few days after her visit and moving things as she suggested, I was sleeping soundly and the pain was gone, hallelujah!
It has saved me a fortune in massages and acupuncture treatments.

Gabi Bruce– Support Team Leader 12WBT-Yoga Teacher – Sydney, Australia

Nicky a huge thank you, I'm finally gaining the balance back in our family life again.
My husband would sleep very shallowly and often wake 1-2 times a night and not be able to settle again and get back to sleep. Due to this, his work was being affected and his stress levels were through the roof. I was getting really worried about him.
After you identified where the Geopathic Stress was in our house, we moved things around according to your suggestions, he is way less stressed and wakes refreshed and even manages to get out for a run before work.

At the dining table where my daughter would never sit still and dinner times were horrible. There were fights for her to sit at the table constantly. She would have a mouthful then get up from the table and run around and not eat properly. The line you found in the dining area ran straight through the chair she always sat at!
I moved the table to the position you suggested and now she is a totally different girl.
She sits to the table during meal times and even if she is finished her meal she will sit and tell us about her day at kindy and partake in the families dinnertime conversation.

Kate –Photographer, Sydney.

Nicky has put a topic that is not well known or understood into an interesting, simple, easy to read book. What if it was that easy? - asks the question we all need to know the answer to, could it be Geopathic stress and it's effects making us sick ? Well Done. A must read.

Shan O'Neil – Hand Analysis- Brisbane, Australia.

I spent 6 months avoiding my new home office. It was beautiful, but whenever I sat at my desk, my creativity was instantly zapped. A friend recommended Nicky to me, and within hours of her visit, I was sitting at my newly positioned desk, filled with energy and newfound focus! I couldn't be happier with the result!

Ani Wilson – Author & International Speaker, Auckland

Before Nicky worked her magic I felt moody, had no energy or motivation and was constantly feeling unwell. My confidence levels had lowered and had less self-esteem. Once Nicky confirmed the bad energy within my workspace I simply moved desks and couldn't believe the difference I felt! I was back to my usual bubbly and ambitious self and my results at work have improved massively.
I would 100% recommend Nicky's services to anybody that is experiencing the above as she has turned it all around for me and I feel great!

Sarah O - Sydney Australia

After not sleeping properly for 6 months, Nicky came in and changed around my room and I haven't slept better. Before she worked her magic, I would get into bed and proceed to lie awake until 3-4am, feeling frustrated. When I'd finally get to sleep I would wake again at 5.30am, not able to get back to sleep.

It was frustrating and was affecting so many other parts of my life including work, family and friendships and my energy and motivation.

Now I get into bed and I feel relaxed and fall to sleep easily. This may not be a great thing, but I actually find it soooo hard to wake up in the mornings, wanting to lie in my comfy bed. This 'comfortable bed', which a few months ago I was cursing as the most horrid bed in the world, and I was about to go out and spend thousands of dollars on a new one! Moreover, when people come to visit they comment on how much better my room looks and feels.

It really has made a difference to my sleeping; my state of calmness and it has had flow on effects in my life in terms of work and relationships.

Erin – Journalist, Sydney Australia

Prior to Nicky's visit into our office I was feeling tired, unmotivated and unwell. I had been moved to a new desk at work and had been continuously ill with women's health issues and spent a lot of time to and from the doctors.

On top of that my sales had slowed and work had gone from being a fun atmosphere, where I wanted to be all the time to something I viewed as a drag.

After Nicky cleared our office and rearranged things away from Geopathic Stress, my luck and most importantly my health changed. I went back to realizing I love my job, my sales went back to being regular and my health has been better than ever.

Also it all happened very quickly after her visit.

<u>Hannah</u> – Manager Sydney.

For a year, I've been taking my 7 year old for chiropractic and podiatry sessions to reduce her discomfort in her left leg. The night after Nicky's visit, I moved my children's bedroom entirely, swapping it with the guest bedroom. That very day whilst at School, my daughter broke her leg. Strangely in her new bedroom she slept soundly and happily with a broken leg anyway.

What was interesting to note however was that although my daughter was supposed to remain in her cast for 5 weeks, and then transfer to a moon-boot for a further 3 weeks, after only 2 weeks her cast was removed and the X-ray showed she had completely healed.

There is no doubt in my mind that although my daughter is an amazing healer naturally, the change in bedrooms was like taking the boulder off her leg finally!

I never mentioned my daughters leg problems to Nicky, but she instantly picked it up in her evaluation. Just amazing! I can't recommend Nicky's work enough!

<u>Ani Wilson</u> – International Speaker – Author

I was having problems sleeping for some time and experienced a funny sensation while lying in bed. As a result of this, I often slept on the couch as I felt more at ease. Through a business introduction, I heard

Nicky speak on Geopathic Stress and was open to the idea of her testing my home for these stress lines.

Nicky established that my side of the bed was directly in line with a geopathic stress energy. I have since moved my bed and have been amazed at how well I am sleeping and feeling.

I would have no hesitation in recommending Nicky as an expert in her field. Can I also add how reasonable priced she was. Thanks for all your help Nicky!

Glen Marsh - Ex Professional Rugby Player

'Such a useful book. It should be on everyone's shelf not just those suffering from the effects of EMF and Geopathic Stress.

Nicky Crocker makes it crystal clear what underlies that suffering-and gives practical advice on how to reverse the situation. Make your home a safer place to be'.

Judy Hall – Author of the Crystal Bibles

& Crystal Prescriptions series.

As you see it may be that EASY!

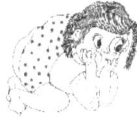

8 CHAPTER EIGHT
HOW DO I FEEL THIS ENERGY!
A GUIDE TO DOWSE.

TOOLS:

Where do I start?

There are so many reference books and advice out there on how to dowse. But the best thing I can do is show you how I learnt and hope you get it.

I'd like to go back to how I first started. The darling 'Ole man - Eric' who first came to my house and identified Geopathic Stress and Underground water in my home was an experienced dowser.

He used a twig! and I wondered what he was doing! How on earth could he 'feel' some underground water under the floor in my bedroom? Firstly I didn't even know there was such a thing. Secondly, how could a 'twig' detect a frequency from some water under the surface of the earth?

Ok, so that is what I first thought when I met the 'dowser' that came into my house to check for Geopathic Stress.

He initially tried to show me how to dowse with his stick or twig, but I couldn't get it.

My son got it immediately.

He was about 10 years old at the time. But when I first tried to do it, I had no idea what I was supposed to be 'feeling'!

So I let it go until the next time I met Eric. He suggested I could use a 'coat hanger'! He had divided one into two 'L' rods.

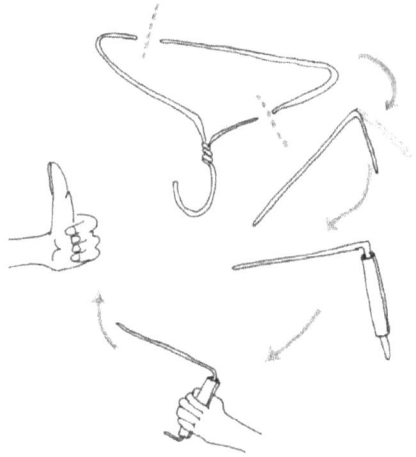

The minute I held them in my hands, I could feel the vibration when I gently walked across the room.

This showed me that even though I couldn't feel the vibration that my son and Eric could feel at my house with the twig, it turned out I just needed a different 'tool' to do it.

So don't give up if the first time you start dowsing you don't get the response you think you should get.

Over 20 years on I have realized there are many different ways of dowsing!

I can now dowse with a stick or twig, metal (either copper or mild steel) a simple coat hanger, and also by simply using my body.

My favourite dowsing rods are retractable ones I ordered from the United States. Tom at Fishercreek hand makes them, (his website is www.dowsingsite.com) they are best because they fold up and retract to a small size. I have them in my bag always and love them, Thanks Tom.

I even carry them when travelling overseas, and often get asked by Customs Officials what they are so great way to start up a conversation about it.

I also occasionally use plastic dowsing rods, which are very effective. They are quite reactive and good for finding water and the depth of things. Some work better for some types of dowsing and some better for other findings.

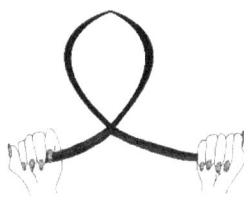

The plastic rods are available on my website or online.

There are other things as simple as twigs from trees. Typically use willow, from a willow tree in the shape of a 'Y'.

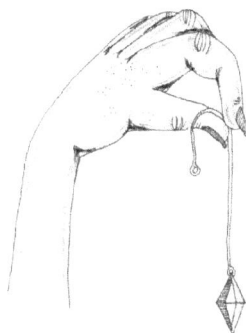

I find the pendulum to be a very sensitive tool and I love using it especially for 'sensitive' work like Distance Dowsing and Map dowsing.

I was given a beautiful diamond necklace for a birthday present and got to choose the one I wanted. I made sure I could use it as a pendulum any time, and anywhere. You will never know when you might need it.

Don't freak out if you cannot 'grasp' any of these tools to start with as your body is the best thing to use if you can train it to work properly. (I'll tell you how to do this soon).

You can use your whole body, your fingers, your tongue, and a whole heap more.

But the most important thing is practice. You may be able to make them move, but can you **understand** the message?

PROTECTION:

Lets start at the beginning.

You will need to get yourself into the right state of mind.

Best way to start is to stand with your hands beside your side, feet at hip width apart and do a couple of big deep breaths.

Start with three deep breaths in through your nose, and out through your mouth.

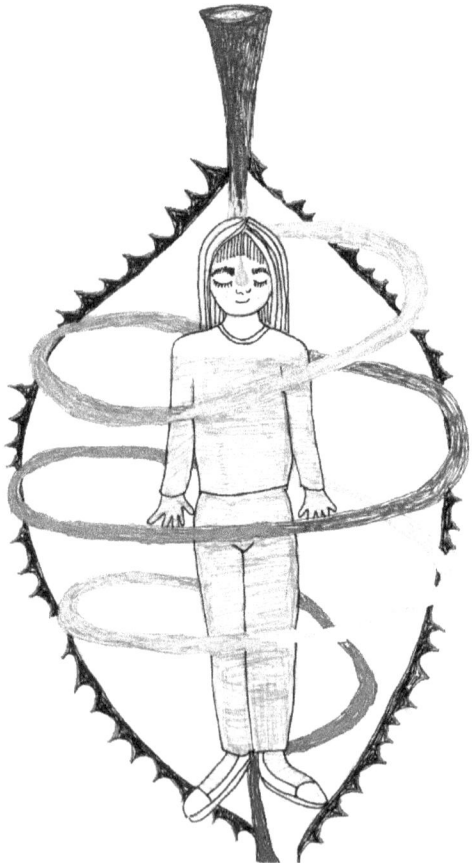

Then I want you to visualize a light coming from high in the heavens, or top of the Universe (whatever suits your soul), it can be whatever colour you like, either white or a multiple of colours. This then needs to 'protect' you so visualize it coming down through your spine and sifting out through your whole body and creating a safe 'bubble' around your body.

The first time you do this take you time and 'feel' it in every part of your body. A bit like an hour-glass filling up with sand from your head to your toes and everywhere in between. After you have done this, visualize it going down through your feet and deep down into the center of the earth for grounding. It can go directly into the core of the earth and then back up like a strong light directly into your heart.

Then say **THANK YOU, THANK YOU, THANK YOU!**

Once you feel that you have completely protected yourself it is then time to ask if you have the skill or ability to actually do the job i.e. dowse. That will come next.

HOW TO DOWSE:

NICKY STYLE

STEP ONE:

All right then, the first thing to do is STOP!

STOP EVERYTHING YOU ARE DOING, AND JUST **STOP**!

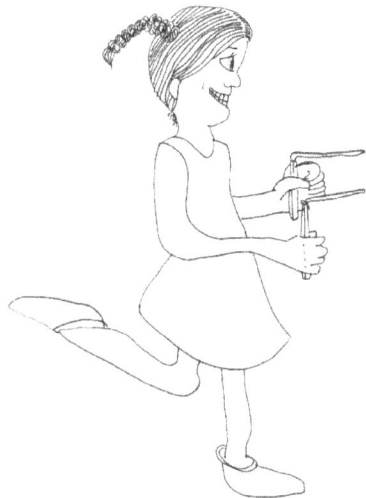

Stop thinking about all the other things you need to do!

Stop worrying if you are getting it right.

Stop, stop, stop, and then BREATHE.

Find yourself a quite place, turn off your phone, and make sure you are not going to be disturbed for a while. Turn the TV off, all music and just STOP.

If you have a whole heap of things whizzing through your head, put them in the 'Beep-It Bucket".

The Beep-it Bucket is a place where you put things that either you don't need to worry yourself over or you can do later. Things that are not your concern, or even things that even though they may be affecting you nothing will change the outcome. Therefore…BEEP IT!

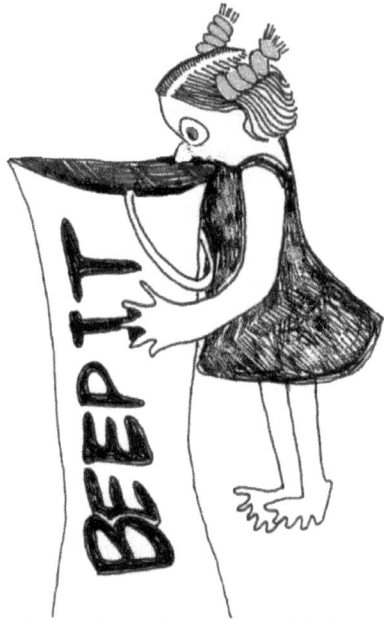

Even things you are worrying about that others may think or say about you. And remember…

"**What someone else thinks of you is none of your business**"!

Therefore the *Beep-it Bucket* is the best place for all those thoughts.

There will always be a 'copy' somewhere in your sub conscious brain for later use if you 'really feel it' or you need to deal with it but for the time being BEEP IT!

STEP TWO:

PROTECTION:

You need to 'protect' yourself because you are going to be asking to 'feel' for the Noxious Earth Energy and the effects of Geopathic Stress or whatever it is you are dowsing for.

These energies ARE 'Noxious' and you do not want to be any more affected than necessary.

If you are asking to dowse to find your keys then it is still a good idea to get that protection.

Follow the steps for protecting yourself as above.

Ok, so now you are protected as previously mentioned, let's get on to the next step.

STEP THREE:

You need to determine what the 'signs' are:

When dowsing generally we start with a YES and NO answers.

This is your body instinctively pushing you forward towards a positive answer or it is pulling you away from a negative answer.

A little bit like if you saw something you really wanted you would head in that direction. Or if there was danger or something that wasn't nice or good for you then instinctively you would pull back away from it.

Like a child in a 'candy store'! You get what I mean.

Occasionally you will get a 'maybe', or ask again. That means your body will most likely do nothing! It will not react in anyway.

It's basically saying "don't treat me like a dummy and ask a sensible question" or it didn't understand the question.

Chances are you have not asked the question correctly. By that I mean you must allow your body to only give a YES or NO response.

So the questions have to be geared that way.

You cannot ask a question like "Should I go left or right"? Or "Is this good for me or not?"

Remember you are asking to get an answer one-way OR the other. Of course you can ask as many questions as you like to get the desired result.

But then is it the 'right' answer if you just keep going until you get the answer you wanted?

Generally when I am using my pendulum, a 'nothing response', will be either no movement, or a movement that goes from 12 to 6 on a clock dial.

I know my YES is clockwise and my NO anti-clockwise.

But you need to find out what 'yours' is! Also occasionally 'check in' even if you have been doing this for a long time, as it may change.

I'll start with your whole body as I do with my clients when I am at their homes. I love to leave them with a gift they can use for the rest of their lives, and this is the same for you.

FIRSTLY:

Stand with your feet shoulder width apart, you may have sat down after I got you to breathe before, but same thing. Three big deep breaths in through your nose and out through your mouth.

Clear your head and then say out loud or to yourself is ok also: "Give me a YES signal"

You are asking your system to give you YOUR, YES signal.

You can use the word POSITIVE instead of 'yes' if you prefer.

Stand quietly and see what happens. You should tip forward

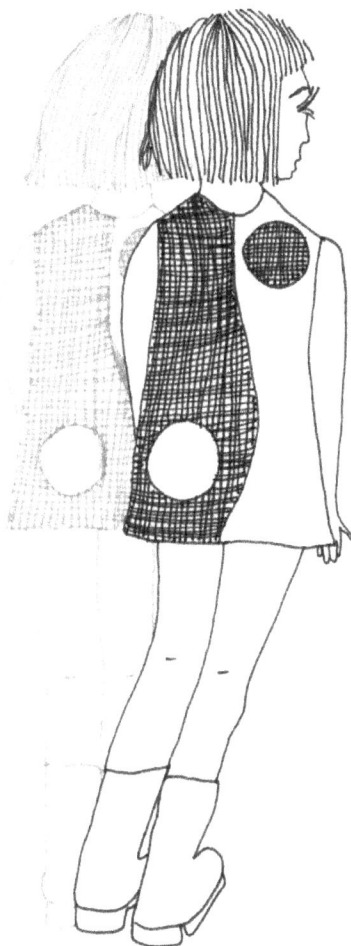

for YES!

But occasionally I have had people sway from side to side or even tip backwards. This reaction could be many things, but usually they are fighting the response and need to practice.

The way to check this is to keep asking questions until you absolutely KNOW beyond any doubt the answers are YES. e.g. "Is my name ......(whatever your name is)? "Am I a Girl/Boy?

Or "Is today Monday"? if it is. Or any other question you choose to ask as long as the only answer could be YES!

Then when you are sure what your YES is, ask your body to "Give me a NO' signal".

Again you should get a signal quite quickly and you will know. Now your body will fall backwards.

To check this, ask a heap of questions that will help you, like is it Monday when in fact it is Wednesday. Or is my name Jill when it is actually Wendy. You get the picture?

Once that is done and you can feel strongly the Yes and No signals ask a question you DON'T know the answer to!

The reason I think you fall forward for YES is because it's a little like when you see something you love and want, you go towards it, and then when you see danger or something you don't like, your body instinctively wants to pull back away from it.

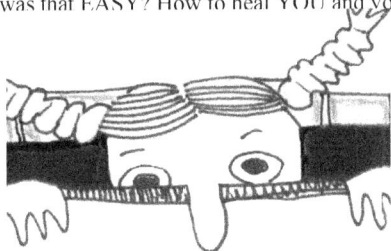

You of course must NOT let *EGO* come into play:

Like saying 'does this boy/girl like me?' especially if you REALLY want the answer to be yes.

Ok so once you know your Yes and No signals, you can start to dowse for other things. So now let's ask permission.

You must ASK! You know the story, 'if you don't ask, you won't receive'!

I tend to ask the first couple of questions all at once, as I am busy and I don't want to waste my valuable time.

I do this every time I dowse.

"CAN I, MAY I, SHOULD I"?

- ✓ **'Can I'?** Means do I have the ability or skill to do the job?

- ✓ **'May I'?** Means, do I have permission from all concerned. The person's house you are dowsing, your house, or whoever it is or wherever it is that you are wanting to know an answer to?

- ✓ **'Should I'?** Is it the right time? Am I in the right state

165

of mind and health? Is it in my (and whoever else is concerned) best interest to do it at this time?

If you get a 'yes', then you can continue.

If you get a no, you have to ask the questions one at a time.

When I am doing dowsing to 'help' other people, most of the time I get a yes.

The only times I get a no, is when I am tired or not well enough to complete it at this time.

I have also had a 'no' when it has been torrential rain and this would have given me a false reading for the client when dowsing to find underground water, as the rain only makes the water appear everywhere and this is not what I want.

I have had a 'no' when I was in a house, trying to check if it was ok to clear the room from 'spirits/entities'.

It turned out the 'entities' weren't ready to talk to me. After I was in the house for about an hour I asked again and I got a yes. Turned out they (the spirits) were not ready to have a conversation with a stranger. I managed to talk to them and later remove them from the house.

I have also had a 'no' if I have had a drink of alcohol.

Always best to be in the 'purest' state of mind.

Now I know not even to try if I feel slightly under the weather in any way. I also don't like dowsing when it's been raining heavily. As I said before, this can affect the reading and won't give an accurate reading, and will magnify the intensity of the GS.

Sometimes it makes it appear everywhere just as it rains on the surface of the earth, it drains down through the ground and if the rain has been constant for days or weeks then the readings are scary, and there is no point passing that on to the client.

Ok, so now we have that out of the way, we have to be VERY clear as to <u>what</u> it is we are dowsing for:

- ✓ Are you looking for underground water?

- ✓ Are you looking for Noxious Earth Energy?

- ✓ Are you looking for any 'harmful energy that may cause illness to the occupants'?

- ✓ Are you looking for a drain, before you dig up the back yard?

- ✓ Or are you looking for your car keys?

Believe me once you practice this you can look for all sorts of things.

But you MUST be very specific.

If I asked to 'feel' the energy in the house I would feel ALL energy and this would not be helpful.

Make sure you are always asking in the positive, and it even helps if you visualize what it is you are trying to find.

That is a bit difficult if you are looking for Geopathic Stress in the form of one of the Earth Grids, (Hartmann or Curry, or Ley lines).

I normally get a feeling, and have also asked my dowsing rods to be specific when they find something. They react differently depending on what it is they find.

For Hartmann they will point in the direction the flow of energy is going. For me the Curry grid point outwards. When it is Underground Water they are pointing inwards.

You will have to 'train' your dowsing rods, or pendulum or whatever tools you use so that you can recognize the answers.

Practice is the only way this will happen.

PRACTICE, PRACTICE, PRACTICE.

'The more you practice the luckier you will get!'

This sign used to be on the wall at my local golf club, but the same rules apply!

Actually to everything!

I have some practice exercises at the back with a page so you can write down some of your own ideas you have come up with.

The exciting thing is it is a work in progress.

I find that with my pendulum, which is very sensitive, I get the answer even before it moves.

The rods are similar.

Now the above instructions apply to whatever tool you use to dowse, so now to the actual TOOLS!

My tools of choice are as already mentioned:

'L' RODS

PENDULUM

'Y' RODS

PLASTIC RODs

YOUR BODY.

Here are the tools in person.

'L' Rods:

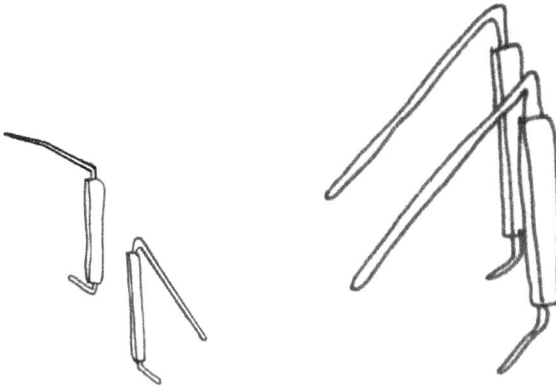

Remember you can make 'L' rods from just opening out a wire coat hanger and cut it at the long end. Undo the 'hook at the top, and open it out so you have two L shape pieces of wire.

Put a 'straw' or you can get a plastic sleeve similar to a straw, and put this on the shorter end of the L Rod, then to stop this from falling off, bend the end up as per image.

Or you can do what I now do and buy some wonderful little retractable L rods online that I can take everywhere with me.

The ones I've mentioned before are handmade by Tom at Fishercreek in the US. (www.dowsingsite.com)

Pendulum

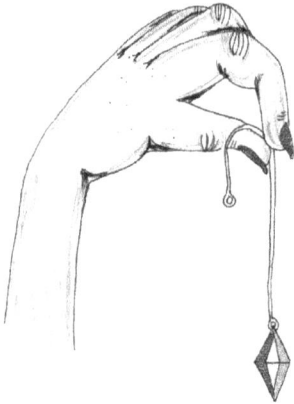

These are fairly self-explanatory.

You can basically use anything that is weighted and attached to a chain or string. It needs to hang with the weight and then move. I have a necklace I love and before I bought it I asked could I use this as a pendulum and got a yes which is perfect, as I always have it on and it has come in handy many times.

Start by asking, "is this pendulum the best, clearest and most accurate pendulum for me to use", or something similar.

With any crystal or natural stone you must 'clear it' of all previous energies. That means whoever has touched it in the process of getting it to you. It could be the person digging it out of the ground or the manufacturer who ground it into the shape it is, or even the shop assistant.

By washing it in the sea I find is best, but salted water is also good if you are not close to the sea. Refer to *Judy Hall's Crystal Bible* books (www.judyhall.co.uk) for more ideas.

When you get your yes you can start dowsing.

Again like the 'L' rods, you will need to be patient and find what your Yes and No is with each tool.

They will vary and that is ok.

With my pendulums, they all seem to go clockwise for yes, and anti-clockwise for no.

It is important to occasionally check this, as previously mentioned as I have known people's answers to change due to certain circumstances. Grief and bereavement can upset the apple cart and change your readings among other things.

Y Rod or Forked stick,

This can be cut directly off a tree. You generally need to be more experienced to use this, but once you get the hang of it, you may find it will turn into your favorite tool. You can find them anywhere, so a good idea to practice with them.

Plastic Rod

This is similar to a Y rod or forked stick and is held in a similar manner to the forked stick.

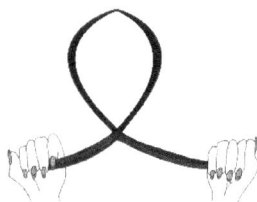

You hold the ends of the rods in your hands, and twist and cross at the same time, which creates a loop with a point at the end.

Then as with all the others, you must find your YES and NO. Once you have done this you can start dowsing.

I find these quite responsive and like having them handy.

They are great for outside as they are fairly heavy duty, and good for outside especially if windy.

See....really EASY!

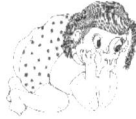

9 CHAPTER Nine
DOWSING TESTS AND EXERCISES
A FUN WAY TO EXPLORE THIS
PHENOMENON

Alrighty then, lets get to the fun bits.

House/Office Dowsing

Choose your 'tool' of choice. I would suggest starting with either L Rods or one of the Y Rods, or a pendulum if that is what you like.

Start at the front door of your house/apartment of office.

Do the deep breathing exercises, including most importantly 'protecting' yourself.

It may take a while to visualize your whole body being protected but the more you practice this, the faster you will get at it.

Then we can start with searching for Geopathic Stress and Noxious Earth Energy.

We want to start with the basic stuff that the 'Earth' creates.

I don't normally like to pre-empt where North is as this could sway my thinking as to which way the rods might move if I walked over a 'Hartman or Curry' grid.

Remember its North South and East West for Hartmann and then diagonal to this for the Curry Grids.

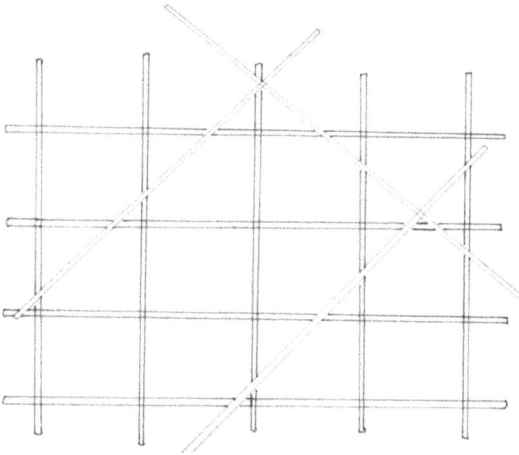

Best thing is to start completely neutral.

Then ASK, what are you looking for?

If you want to start looking for Geopathic Stress in your home try this;

"Show me any Noxious Earth Energy, Geopathic stress, or Underground Water that may be affecting anyone who lives in this house, now"!

Then start walking slowly with your rods in your hands. If you have a plastic sleeve (or similar like my retractable rods), you can hold them as tight as you like, because it will not stop the rods from moving.

If you are using L rods without a sleeve, then you need to hold them lighter as if you are you are holding a tray of eggs.

Firm but you don't want to break them. They of course need to move slightly in your hands so they can turn when necessary.

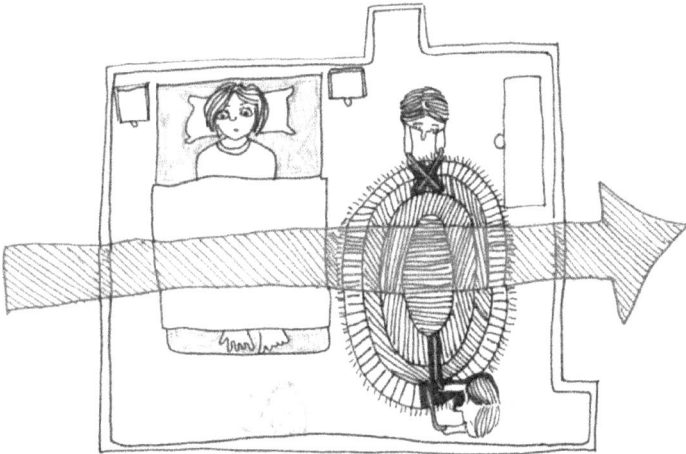

Now GRID through the space you are working on. That means go left to right and right to left, then opposite to that so you cover every space in the room.

You will need to go in each direction so you can find any of the lines that may be affecting the place you are dowsing.

Once you have walked through the whole area you will get a picture of what is going on.

Before you start it can be a good idea to draw a basic plan of the house, and mark out where the lines are crossing each room.

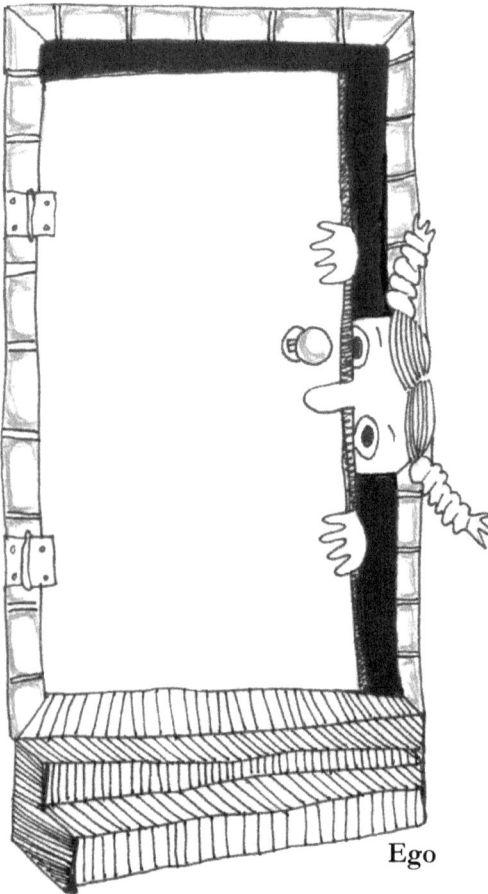

Continue drawing the line as if it continues straight in the direction it is pointing, through the walls. Then when you go into the other rooms, see if the line you find in that rooms lines up with the other one.

I always try to make the furniture not a feature so I am not being affected by where the furniture is. You know there is a bed and maybe there is a problem but don't let EGO over ride your judgment.

Ego

If there is Geopathic Stress crossing a bed, chair or couch, or any other place where you spend time stationary then you need to know where it is.

One of the things I feel is there is an edge to these lines. Whether they are one of the GRIDs (Hartmann, Curry) or Underground Water, there is a definite edge to it. You need to work out exactly where this edge is because if you are off it then you should be ok. If you're not off it, then ...that's a whole different story.

Now let's look for something else. Dowsing gives us the opportunity to explore the world.

Your imagination is literally the only thing that is holding you back.

Say you want to find your keys or a lost ring! Anything is possible.

The most important thing you must remember is to be very clear as to what your YES and NO is.

Then you need to make sure you leave EGO at the door!

Then off you go. Here are a few tests for you to try.

Get someone to hide something, maybe a piece of metal, a coin or anything in the house.

Then you need to 'tune in' to what it is and ask your dowsing tool, to direct you to where it is.

Make sure your questions are direct and to the point and they must have a clear YES, NO or Direction answers.

You can't say, " Is it left or right"? Or is it in this room or that one"? Ask each one separately.

The fun thing is the more you practice the better you will get at it.

Use a pack of cards, and lay out 3 cards. Then get your pendulum or dowsing rods, and first ask if it's a red card, (Y or N?). Once you have worked out if it is red or black then you need to ask, depending on if it is red (hearts or diamonds), or if it is black (spades or clubs) then once you have decided which suit you think it is, then ask "Is it a picture card"? (Y or N), and you can slowly determine what the card is.

You can always just start with deciding the suit and not go down to as low as the exact the number.

This is a good way of building your confidence.

But it is something you can work on, and certainly don't get yourself all worked up if you get it wrong. There is no such thing as wrong with dowsing. It is more about understanding the answers you are receiving according to the questions you have asked.

It's like riding a bike and practice is paramount. It is a total learning curve recognizing what your signals are with your choice of dowsing tool, and taking 'Mr./Miss Ego' out of the equation.

You need to recognize this new language you are learning and most importantly listen!

Listen to your gut and guidance system and of course finally...

Don't give up!

WHAT ELSE IS DOWSING GOOD FOR?

What if I have no tools with me?

Ok, now lets try some other fun dowsing test.

You can pretty much dowse for ANYTHING!

You can ask questions that you don't know the answers to. Probably not a good idea to ask what the lotto numbers are, but you never know your luck in a big city!

But I do believe the possibilities are limitless.

Now the question is 'what if I left my tools elsewhere and I need to ask a question'?

Easy, use your body!

For a start, the tools previously mentioned are only an 'antenna' to your body anyway, so if you can use your body without the tools, then you are not reliant on them.

There are lots of things you can do, but the one I love the most is using your whole body as previously mentioned in the last chapter.

Once you have mastered using your whole body, with the 'sway test' don't forget you must always remember to ask the 3 important questions first.

"Can I, May I, Should I"?

Then go for it!

- ✓ Ask away and have a ball.

- ✓ You could be at the supermarket and want to know if that avocado is the best one for you to buy.

- ✓ You don't really want to get your pendulum or dowsing rods out so you can just quickly ask in your head and see what happens.

- ✓ Another one I really like is I use my fingers. I can even use this when I'm driving, even with both hands still on the steering wheel.

- ✓ Use the opposite hand to the one you write with, and put the first finger up and over the middle finger.

- ✓ Like you have 'crossed your fingers' but make sure that the first finger is on top of the middle one.

- ✓ Then do the same thing and ask for your 'yes'. With this one, when you ask, you try to pull your top finger down and off the middle finger.

My 'yes' is it sticks. I am unable to get the top finger off of bottom finger. For a 'no' it slips off easily.

If you can't grasp this one, you can use two fingers. Use your thumb and first fingers on both hands and create a circle with each but linked.

Then ask for your yes and no again one at a time. For me on this one my yes sticks closed and I can't break the loops. And 'no' will break easily.

This is another cool dowsing 'tool' you can use when you are out and about. Again like all dowsing it is practice that makes it reliable and a lot more fun.

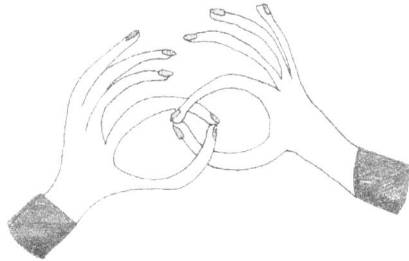

There is one more I will mention, and this is using your tongue. You need to have your tongue in a neutral position in your mouth, with your mouth closed and jaw relaxed. (Just floating in the middle).

Ask for a 'Yes' and typically it will lift to the roof of your mouth. And a 'No' should drop to the bottom of your mouth.

This is another cool one if you practice it and know what your Y & N are. You can do it anywhere.

Very handy!

Now go and play and practice!

SOME WAYS TO PRACTICE:

Use whichever tool, (Pendulum, L-Rods, Y' stick or body) that you feel most comfortable, or try all of them.

If you have a pet, a dog, cat, fish or bird, hold the pendulum or 'L' rods over the pet and ask "Is this…..fill in the blank"?

2. Hold it over some food that you want to know is ok for you to eat? But remember you must ask, and it can only have a Yes or No answer like "Is this healthy for me to eat"?

3. Try asking about some food that is an unhealthy option and see what the answer is?

4. You can test the plants in your garden and ask if they are doing ok, or do they need anything? "Do you need fertilizer"? Do you need more water? Or less water? Get the idea?

5. Try getting someone to hide some things and using your tools of choice, find them. Remember the more questions you ask the closer you will get. It is also about the 'quality' of your questions.

I heard of a good idea when I was learning and it was to place a large photo of a body of water, a picture of a lake or river under a large mat. Best if you get someone else to place it under or you will know where it is. Then ask to find the water.

The same can apply if you live in a multi-level house or apartment. You can get someone to put a glass of water downstairs in an area, and you need to find it.

My children wanted to test my Dad and hid an avocado in the lounge. He found it.

I have used it to find all sorts of things including lost jewelry. The sky is the limit!

Just remember you should only ever use dowsing for good. Don't think you can use it to find the lotto numbers. (not that, that wouldn't be good, just not right!)

Write down your fun EASY ideas you've practiced!

WRITE DOWN YOUR PRACTICE IDEAS & TESTS HERE OR IN A SPARE NOTEBOOK:

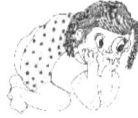

10 CHAPTER TEN
WHAT ELSE CAN HELP?
ENERGY BOMBS & CRYSTALS ETC

I have a product called an "Energy Bomb™" which is a small handmade ceramic pot filled with minerals and crystals that work to block and alleviate the effects of Geopathic Stress, including a calming from the effects of EMR and EMF's.

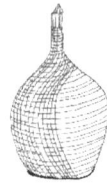

Check **out Judy Hall's new book "Crystal Prescriptions Volume 3'** (www.judyhall.co.uk) Including all her other amazing books on Crystals, for some of the amazing crystals we used and many others that help alleviate and soften the effects of Geopathic Stress, and Electromagnetic radiation and fields.

These are getting more and more prevalent with everyone having a mobile phone. Everywhere in my country there are cell towers, if they are not stand alone ones on every corner, they have been hidden on top of buildings and some not even so hidden anymore.

Some of the crystals I love are Black Tourmaline, Amazonite, Amethyst, Brown Jasper, Flint, Granite, Smoky Quartz, Kunzite, Labradorite, Sodalite, Shungite and Orgonite to name but a few.

(Judy's book is full of lots of helpful information). Thank you Judy for your informative books. They have been a godsend over the years. She has many in her library and most are available on her website (www.judyhall.co.uk) or on Amazon.

In my experience however I always feel it is better to be OFF this energy called Geopathic Stress or any other noxious earth energy if at all possible. I myself have my Energy Bombs close to where I am spending time stationary i.e. bed, couch and desk. But I also know that where I am sitting or sleeping is clear of GS, and the minimum amount of EMF's/EMR's.

If GS is strong enough to be detected high up in apartment blocks and I have found it as high as 43 stories up in Martin Place in Sydney, and there are reports that is has been found as high as 100 stories up in apartment/office buildings, then why would you want to risk it?

The other thing that needs to be considered is if you are in an apartment building, and the people below you are being affected then their negative energy can affect you also. (Sick Building Syndrome).

Obviously there are going to be cases when it is almost impossible to move the bed and then you need to consider other things.

Maybe you can move the bed, (if it's on wheels or not too

heavy) before you go to sleep and move back in the morning.

Believe me, the difference in a good night sleep verses sleep deprivation, is enormous. It also has 'flow-on' effects on the rest of your life.

I have tried all the other options like putting cork under the bed as was suggested to me many years ago by a dowser, but I didn't feel any difference. There is also the idea to 'copper-rod' the house or the lines of GS in your house. Again I had several experts come and do this to my house, but it had either no affect, or one time it turned my house into a 'pressure cooker'!

Even my darling 'skeptical' husband could feel it. We released the copper rods and it was like a whirlwind inside the house. I have tried many other different ways of copper rodding and even using other 'energetic' treatments like Reiki, NLP and Kinesiology to change the energy from noxious to positive. This definitely can work for short periods. You can dowse for how long it will last for. Sometimes I've had it up to 18months or two years.

As we know the Earth is always moving, and many places even if they cannot feel it have earthquakes or at certain times will have extreme rainfall or even drought. This can also affect the lines of energy. I have been back years later to client's homes and still found the GS in exactly the same place when I have referred back to their plan.

If you can't move the bed, couch or chair to a location you are happy with you can always try the previous options and see if you notice a difference.

Make sure however you know what you are doing, and you have 'checked-in' with your system to make sure you have permission, and you are not opening a can of worms.

I believe if you try to block the energy or re-direct it, you are perhaps sending it to your neighbour or to someone else, and it might make them sick. This is not good karma.

If you tried to block a river or creek, it could either over flow or find another way out. So instead of 'knowing' where this energy is you create a monster and it turns into several lines.

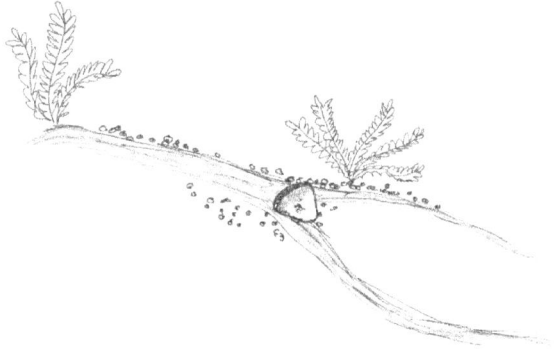

There is a great easy test an amazing dowser in Ireland (Brendan Murphy www.positiveenergy.ie) told me about. This is a good way to tell if you have GS under your bed.

It's the 'Tin-foil' or aluminum foil test.

Place tinfoil, shiny side facing down, under your mattress or bed. This will block the noxious energy.

But do not leave it any longer than 10days (2 weeks) as it will also block the 'good energy' as well.

If after the two weeks you notice a difference and have better sleep at night, there is a good chance you need to relocate your bed.

NEXT STEP: - TRY IT OUT!

Now you need to find where it is in your bed as this is where you spend time stationary, so get your dowsing rods out, the ones you like or feel the most comfortable with.

I like my 'L' rods for this, as they are not only very reactive but also show me the direction the line is going.

You might find it is only on one side of the bed, and you can safely move the bed to one side or another. It may be crossing your pillows and head so you could move your bed away from the wall. If it is crossing diagonally across the bed, then it gets a bit tricky if you have a small room.

If you have two lines 'knotting' on your bed, then this is of a big concern.

'Knots' are dangerous if you are spending time **stationary** on them. To be fair even just a line of GS energy can be dangerous, but knots are worse.

Remember the statistics I mentioned previously where up to 80% of people diagnosed with chronic illnesses are found to be sleeping on Geopathic Stress zones. It will more than likely be on one of these knots.

No 'knots' in the bed!

What if it was that easy?

I have these cool little cards called Neutralise Cards. They also have the healing modality called 'Sanjeevini' infused into them. They are magic. They neutralise the noxious energy, but I have many wonderful stories of them ridding all sorts of other noxious stuff from people's lives.

You just carry them in your pocket or bra. One client calls it her 'bra-card'! These are available on my website (www.clearenergyhomes.com/services). Look for Neutralise Cards.

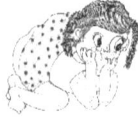

11 CHAPTER ELEVEN

CAN YOU BE YOUR OWN HOUSE DOCTOR?

WHAT TO LOOK FOR

The power within!

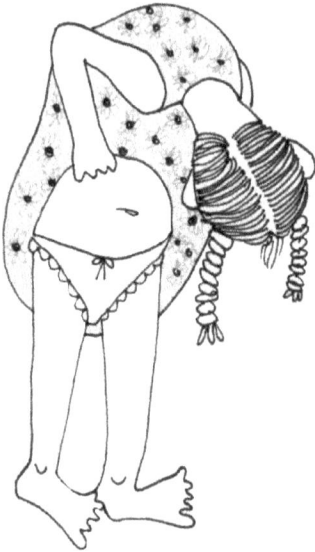

Ok, firstly I want to state very clearly I am not a Doctor. Nor do I in anyway say that you should not take the advice of your own doctor, Specialist or other medical professional.

What I am saying is:

LISTEN TO YOUR GUT!

We are all so quick to believe anything and everything that a professional tells us because they have a certificate!

No one has more knowledge about YOUR body than YOU, so just listen.

Sure there are so many questions and so many possible answers, and sometimes we just don't want to listen or don't understand the answers when we get them. It can certainly be very overwhelming. But if you give your body the chance, and truly listen, you will hear the answers.

You know what I mean! How many times have you had a message from your 'gut' or 'system' or whatever you want to call it and it was bang on!

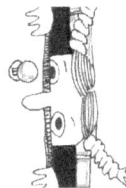

The biggest trick is to get rid of little ole EGO!

He (I say he, because to me, it feels like a male), or you may feel a she, or even no gender) has the knack of tricking you into believing things that your brain might want you to do or think.

The part of your body, that is educated and listens to what is written out there or you have learned over the years. Not the inner wisdom that only your body can tell you.

By using dowsing to discover this voice inside you, you open up a whole world of discovery.

What if self-healing is just the ability to trust your gut?

Ask your body;

- ✓ What is this pain?

- ✓ Why do I have it?

- ✓ What is in there?

- ✓ Where in my body is the pain?

- ✓ Is this the center of it?

- ✓ What is it saying?

Sure it may say take a pill to get rid of it but if that means it is going to come back again and again. Do you really want that?

Some of the answers you get may be so simple.

Some of them you may not like because you already knew the answer, but you don't want to do that. Whatever 'that' is.

Chances are the answers are in you. But we have come to a space in time where we want a 'quick' answer. We want quick results even if they are harming our bodies. Quick painkiller. Pain gone.

If your body has pain, it is trying to tell you something.

LISTEN!

Get your pendulum out (or just your fingers or whole body if that is good for you) and ask away.

Write down a list of questions like:

- ✓ "Are these pills (or other medication/supplement etc.)

adding positive value to my life?

- ✓ "Are they in my best and highest interest"?

- ✓ "Is this exercise the best for my body"?

- ✓ "How many glasses of water do I need to drink in a day?" Then count 1, 2, 3, 4…Keep going until you get a yes and see where it stops.

You literally can ask your body all the important questions, and take the guessing out. Your body might say you only need 5 glasses of water per day, and that might be ok for your body. Or it might say you need 15 glasses.

Again it is all about asking what is good for you.

Don't forget you must always ask the question so it can only have a 'yes or no' answer.

If you ask something like, "Should I take these supplements"?

You could easily get and Y or N but the thing is, 'should' is very ambiguous.

You could easily take them and they may not have any benefit either way, but 'should' is not asking 'Are they going to add value to my life'?

Are they going to improve my bodily function, and help whatever part of my body they have been purchased for?

A better way to ask would be…

"Are these …(fill in the gap)… the best and highest good for my life right now?

Do you see?

You must make the questions VERY specific to what it is you want to know at this time.

The question and answer you need may be different tomorrow, or in the future. You may need some supplement or medication today, but your body may heal or outgrow the requirements and then you won't need it. I think it's a good practice to get into occasionally just checking are these still for your best and highest good.

I used to work in Australia for a company where I was in and out of Pharmacies all day every day, and used to see the customers with this huge pile of prescribed pills. I remember saying to a man one day who had the biggest pile ever and I just said "I'm sorry'!

He turned around and said 'what for'? I said "you must be very sick and I'm sorry'! He said "oh no, I don't even know what most of these are for but I think this one causes a side effect so I need that one, then that one causes another side effect so I need that one and so it goes on"!

I was gob-smacked, he had no idea what he was taking and blindly believed he needed them because that's what someone had told him.

If he had the skills you now do, he could have 'tuned in' and gone through his medication and at least asked his 'system' or body what exactly it needs.

By all means then go back to the Doctor and say, "Do I really need to take these"? (The ones identified by dowsing that you think you don't need) and see what they say.

Chances are they may screw up their face, and say of course you need them, but they may also say, you could give it a go without it and see how you go if it is not life threatening to go without. Or they may suggest it's time to be retested and see if anything has changed?

My dear ole Dad does this all the time. He dowses over the medication he is prescribed and decides if he needs it or not. If he doesn't he chooses not to take it. He's nearly 82 and doing great.

We are all so easily lead by what we are told, and the things we read or taught verbatim at school, and especially what we see on TV.

If it's on TV it must be real - right?

What is REAL is the gift YOU have inside yourself. Your inner wisdom, your higher self, your Guidance system, Gut instinct, God, Grace, the Universe or whatever name you choose to give it.

It is the gift we are all born with and sadly many of us lose as adults as society tell us otherwise. This is not their fault as they just didn't know either.

Choose to listen to your gut, anyway you can!

Turn on YOUR inner knowing!

See how it helps you live and
move forward for a happier,
healthier more outstanding future
YOU.

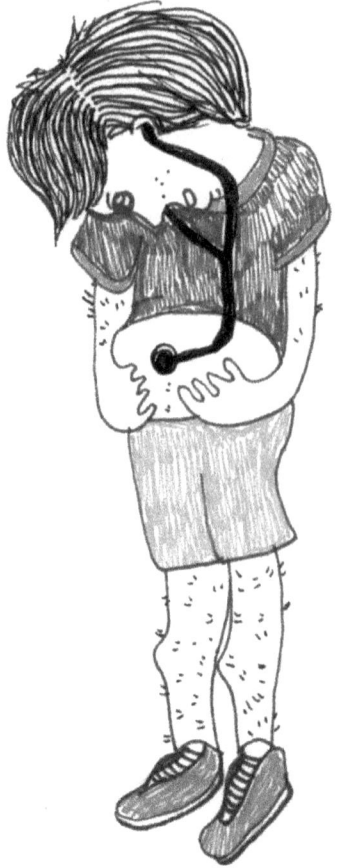

What if it was that EASY?

FREQUENTLY ASKED QUESTIONS

1. How wide spread is Geopathic Stress? Isn't everybody affected one way or another?

A: Geopathic Stress is part of Nature. It helps to disintegrate life forms and accelerates the rotting process. In this function it plays an essential part of the life cycle (brings back 'dust to dust'). However not everything in nature is made to keep us young and healthy. There are lots of poisonous plants; animals and toxic materials so stay away from those! A healthy body generally bounces back after exposure to stress and especially Geopathic Stress.

2. Could my whole house be affected?

A: There are lines all over the world and some can be as close together as a few meters, but generally they are not very wide so there is usually a place you can move your bed to. Even half a metre can make a difference.

3. Does it affect Children?

A: Yes if affects children more than adults especially new born babies and indeed unborn babies. Tests carried out by the *Dulwich Health Society in the* UK found that 80% of Cot Deaths were linked to sleeping above a Geopathic Stress zone.

4. How do I know if I've been affected?

A: The most common symptoms are tiredness in the mornings, inability to sleep, tossing and turning during the night, waking regularly anywhere from 10pm-3am. Inability to heal, or reoccurring illnesses or disease in a particular location in the body. e.g. constant neck ache, or back ache. You tend to blame the bed or pillow, but it could be the location of them. Geopathic Stress could be causing the irritation.

5. If I'm affected, what do I do?

A: The first and cheapest option is to move your bed or chair at work. If you want to be sure get a reputable dowser to come and check your home/office or read this book and practice. Or contact me at www.clearenergyhomes.com

6. How long before I'd notice something if I WAS affected by GS?

A: If you are sensitive you may notice it quite quickly. You may sit in a chair and feel a heavy feeling, or a feeling of 'disease' but not quite understand what it is. You may notice a headache come on quite quickly or a tingling and irritability. Or it could take 5 years or more if you have become immune to it and just brush it off as 'growing old' or just 'life'!

The longer you are exposed to Geopathic Stress for long periods at a time (i.e. your bed, sofa/couch, or office) you can become used to the irritable feeling, and just accept it as the norm. But by then your immune system has been compromised so other more serious illnesses and disease take hold.

7. What if both my cat and dog sleep on my bed?

A: I have mentioned before that in the old days they use to use a dog to sit and stay in a location for 10 minutes unrestrained to check if it was clear of Geopathic Stress and safe for humans to spend time, or even build a bedroom. A

Dog is like a human in the fact the GS zone irritates them as well so would move away or be irritable if placed on one of these locations. However a cat is drawn to the frequency of Geopathic Stress. So if you have a place in your home that has a line or 'knot' (where two lines cross) of this energy in your home, cats are attracted to it. That is to say, as long as it is not where it is nice and sunny and you are also, then chances are they are attracted to that location because there is also GS present. They are not attracted because it is 'negative or noxious', but the frequency of energy creates a heat and they are drawn to that. Just like all things in nature, we have to have Yin and Yang, right and wrong, good and bad and up and down, so we have to have things that thrive in Geopathic Stress. For example many plants used as medicinal herbs grow in these areas, as they need the qualities to help heal.

Now the reason you dog and cat may be sleeping on the same bed is that there could be a line of geopathic stress on one side of the bed, the side the cat likes, and nothing on the side that the dog likes.

8. We have a history of cancer in our family, should I be afraid too?

A: Let me make it very clear, that I am NOT a doctor, so I cannot give any medical advice and never will. I try to support medical treatments through energetic measures. In a case of cancer it is very often overseen that the illness occurs because of a specific cause, more likely a combination of causes. To deal with the symptom (e.g. a tumor) is necessary, but should not distract us from looking for causes at the same time otherwise the cancer will come back. Family history often indicates common patterns in living space, food and nutrition and lifestyle habits. I recommend we should consider these things.

1. German studies since the late 1920's show that geopathic zones are practically always found in cases of cancer. In my opinion it is essential to change the sleeping location and/or shield the space with energetic measures.

2. Nutritional patterns of overly acidic food, sugars, sodas, alcohol, junk food and the lack of essential nutrients (minerals, vitamins, amino acids, essential fatty acids), lack of anti-oxidants.

3. An accumulation of stress from personal trauma, stress at work or even long periods of tense economic situations including long periods of time on geopathic stress.

In saying all that, I have also had clients with lung cancer that never smoked, or liver cancer and never been heavy drinkers. Also melanoma in places the sun doesn't get to.

9. If I have been affected, can I get it out of my system?

A: Yes. Once your body comes off Geopathic Stress and you are spending the majority of your time such as your bed or office GS Free your body will start to heal itself again and your immune system can begin to strengthen. Obviously you must be patient as it can take at least 6 to 8 weeks especially if you have been affected for a long time. Some people have been exposed to regular bouts of GS for most of their life. You must of course also continue with the other important things like regular exercise, good healthy food, regular rest and water.

ABOUT THE AUTHOR

NICKY CROCKER

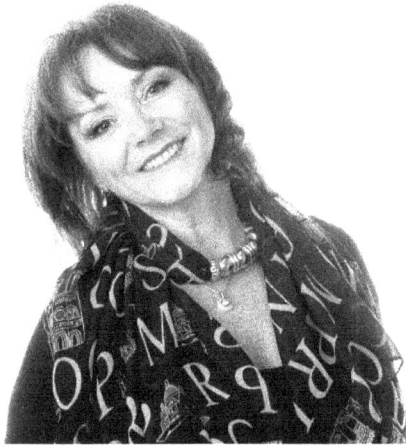

Nicky was born in the small town of Hororata in Mid Canterbury, New Zealand. Her family moved regularly during her early years, and she was inspired and influenced heavily by rural New Zealand through the many small towns she lived in during her childhood where she experienced the best of kiwi country living.

She went to 8 different schools, which meant she was always the new kid at school. It was either sink or swim being constantly the 'new girl' - so she swam. As an adult she still loves to swim, loves the water and as is always living not far from the sea.

Ironically water would prove to become an important part of

her life going forward, not just drinking it.

As a child, Nicky remembers her Grandfather searching for water with some old sticks, but never thought much about it until some 30 odd years later.

Diagnosed with 'chronic arthritis' in her feet, she was introduced to a 'dowser' who checked her home for underground water and Geopathic Stress. She never expected that the extreme pain in her feet was caused by the location of her bed, which was being aggravated by the underground water and Earth's Magnetic fields that were in her bedroom.

After years wondering what was going on, Nicky was doing everything she could to keep healthy with regular exercise, massage, reflexology, and a sensible diet. So why were her feet so sore? She bought the best quality running shoes and had them fitted by the professionals but was still in constant pain.

She assumed that age was a factor and this is what you have to expect, as you get older – Right?

After a second painful cortisone injection into the joint of her toe, and regularly taking painkillers to the point it gave her a stomach ulcer which required treatment, she decided there must be another way.

As luck (or guidance from The Universe) would have it, she had a Vega Test conducted by Gary King D.Ac at Mairangi Bay, Auckland. Gary is a naturopath and uses this machine to help define issues initially unrecognized.

This is a device that does a form of electro-acupuncture. Proponents claim this device can diagnose allergies and other illnesses, including arthritis and Geopathic Stress.

It picked up that not only was Geopathic Stress affecting her, but also her body was like a 100-year-old mushroom. This meant was she being affected by GS, to the point that internally it had gone mouldy and turned into fungus – Oooowwwww!

She immediately set out to find a dowser who could help. Remember this was before the Internet, so not as easy to find as it is today. You couldn't just go and 'Google it'!

She was advised to find a person who was not only a dowser with the ability to find oil and water, but could also advise how it can affect your health.

She located a respected dowser who as a result of an accident many years earlier had his powers of healing enhanced. He was very intuitive to Noxious Earth Energies including identifying how Geopathic Stress affects the body and your home.

After soaking up all the knowledge this 'ole dowser' had to offer, she set about dowsing everything and everybody's homes she knew. Initially only dowsing for friends and family, Nicky quickly recognized the links with illness and injury where they were sleeping or working.

How was she going to spread the word?

Everyone said it couldn't be done. No one had heard of Geopathic Stress.

- ✓ **"I can't move my bed",**

- ✓ **"I've never heard of this before",**

- ✓ **"My house is too small",**

- ✓ **"I don't have the room to move anything",**

- ✓ **"I like it the way it is",**

- ✓ **"I'd rather not know",**

- ✓ **"If it is so bad for us, how come no one has told me about this before now?" etc. etc.…**

The only way she thought she could get the word out was one person at a time. With her training in Reiki, Reflexology, and interest in Naturopathy, Kinesiology, Meditation, EFT/ Tapping, Feng Shui, Dowsing and many other self-healing modalities, she has developed a strong intuition for Geopathic Stress, EMF/EMR and dowsing.

With this 6th (has even been described as our 7th) sense, she can detect where GS is in your home and office or any other place you spend long periods of time.

Whether she gets to visit you in person, and she loves to travel or does it by 'Distance Dowsing', she has accurately identified the Geopathic Stress in people's homes all over the world including New Zealand, Australia, England, Ireland, Scotland, Germany, Italy, Austria, Switzerland, South Africa, Singapore, Brazil, Chile, USA, China and Russia.

Nicky's goal is to educate and teach people to recognize this 'energy' themselves? To know that when something is not right and before you rush to the doctor, to tune in. When did this happen?

Obviously if it's an accident, go STRAIGHT to the Doctor

or Hospital. But if it's an illness that may have slowly crept up on you then you need to know the tools she has taught you in this book.

These Earth's energies and magnetic fields are everywhere and they are so important for life as we know it and we need them however ..

Just like we need the sun for our very existence, if you stay out in it too long you will get burnt!

Tune in to your body's wisdom, listen to your 'gut' and see if you can help heal yourself and your home! At the very least it will help to provide a better understanding for you and your family.

What if it was that EASY?

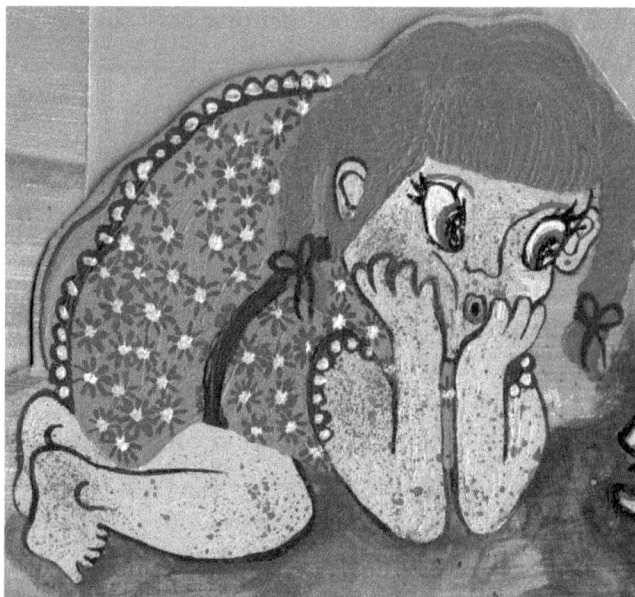

WHAT IF IT WAS THAT EASY?

www.ingramcontent.com/pod-product-compliance
Lightning Source LLC
Chambersburg PA
CBHW062222270326
41930CB00009B/1827